TALK YOURSELF SLIM WITH
THE DR. ROCKET'S
SELF-CHATTER
DIET

BEHAVIOUR FOCUSED WEIGHT-LOSS SUCCESS

TALK YOURSELF SLIM WITH

THE DR. ROCKET'S
SELF-CHATTER
DIET

BEHAVIOUR FOCUSED WEIGHT-LOSS SUCCESS

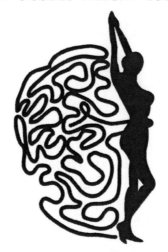

JOHN RICHARDSON

BEHAVIOURAL WEIGHT-LOSS CONSULTANT / NBW-LP

Matador
9 Priory Business Park
Kibworth Beauchamp
Leicestershire LE8 0RX, UK
Tel: (+44) 116 279 2299
Fax: (+44) 116 279 2277
Email: books@troubador.co.uk
Web: www.troubador.co.uk/matador

ISBN 978 1783063 369

British Library Cataloguing in Publication Data.
A catalogue record for this book is available from the British Library.

Typeset in Aldine401 BT Roman by Troubador Publishing Ltd
Printed and bound in the UK by TJ International, Padstow, Cornwall

Matador is an imprint of Troubador Publishing Ltd

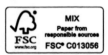

*This book is dedicated to my grandfather
Mr J. A. Laundon who knew all the secrets
of life and longevity and he himself proved
their worth. Also the National Association
of Holistic Hypnotherapists (NAHH) and
the British Academy of Hypnosis (B.A. Hyp)
because without their passing of knowledge
this book could have never been written.*

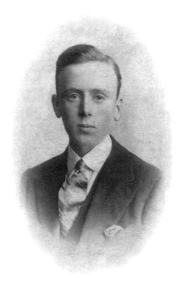

Disclaimer

The information in this book is the sole view and opinion of the author and intended as a reference volume only. Any decisions you make about your lifestyle are your own and you remain wholly responsible for any decisions and action you take. This book is not intended to be a substitute for proper medical attention and advice. If in any doubt, please contact your family doctor or local medical centre.

CONTENTS

INTRODUCTION

MR JOHN RICHARDSON AND
TALK YOURSELF SLIM WITH
THE SELF-CHATTER DIET

*'Life should be lived instinctive and natural, but we
continue to fight, trying to control nature. Eating and
drinking should be as instinctive as breathing, we are
not and never will be qualified to change or modify
natures original product.'*

J. Arthur Laundon, 1909-2000

From when I was a small boy, I watched the constant
battle my mother fought with her weight and how
effortlessly my grandfather had always remained
slim. He was a natural healthy weight all throughout his
life. I became fascinated with these two people, so similar
and yet very different. My grandfather would eat a wide
variety of foods from salads to the traditional full English

breakfast and still his weight never changed. My mother, on the other hand, that is a very different story. She attended every diet club she could find, going from one to the next, then back to the first, but sadly never did find the answers she was looking for. The one thing I did notice was that my grandfather would often leave food and when asked by the inquisitive child why, his reply would always be, "I know when I have had enough." It's now obvious that my mother didn't! I discovered early in my life the true causation of obesity; that learnt behaviours or habitual auto-behaviours, along with corresponding triggered associations formed from fallacious beliefs, result in the change or modification of the original primal instinct, otherwise know as the Master Programme, to eat when hungry and stop when satisfied. Today the majority of eating is done for reasons mostly other than hunger.

I asked my mother one lunchtime as she sat down to eat, "Are you really hungry and I mean really hungry?" She said, "Not really." "Then why are you eating?" I asked. "Because it's lunch time," was her reply, and to her this was a very logical and obvious answer to a question she had never thought to ask. My mother was a fantastic cook but also a fantastic feeder with regimented meals, and the people she fed were expected to empty their plates. As often as I could I would escape my mother's forced-feeding regime. If I had my way, I chose to eat at my grandparents where I could eat as much or as little as I liked. I found this freedom a relief and with age and awareness would often say to my mother, "I'm sure that forcing a child to eat when they're not hungry is child abuse." Not only does it cause pain at the time, but forcing a child to eat also permanently damages him or her by reprogramming their primal instincts, the Master Programme, and inflicting the misery of a lifetime spent in the continual company of obesity. To my mother this was just ridiculous. My mother would ask, "Do you want seconds?" But before you could answer you would find that seconds were on your plate with the full expectation that they would be eaten. As a child I would often be taken to the doctor's by my worried mother, who firmly believed that I was not eating enough to keep a sparrow alive. The doctor would always tell her that, while perhaps I wasn't eating the amount of food she expected me to, I was eating the amount of food I needed. "A child will never starve," he would say. "I promise you he will eat when he is hungry." Dr Mitchell was an ex-army doctor who knew all the secrets of natural instinctive eating.

My grandfather would often say as my mother returned

home from her habitual Wednesday night diet club meeting, "I wouldn't have someone telling me what I could and couldn't eat." Then he would say to me. "You know how they fatten a pig don't you? Feed it! If you, Johnny-boy, start becoming overweight, then let me know. I will pop round and stitch your mouth up, because it's what you're putting into your mouth that is causing the problem." He actually saw this as caring and loving advice because he had seen the pain and misery his own daughter had endured due to nothing more than being overweight. He knew how different it could have actually been. So the pain of stitching his grandson's mouth up would bear no comparison to the pain suffered living a lifetime of obesity. As a child and until the age of twenty-six, my mother was a very natural and healthy weight, slim in fact. Learnt behaviours or habitual auto-behaviours, along with all their corresponding triggered associations, and the constant yo-yo effect caused by the same diet/slimming clubs my mother has sought for help, took my mother's weight to the opposite extreme. She is one of the many soldiers in an army of millions fighting the Weight War; for some I fear, a battle that will never be won.

In my mother's mind feeding was caring. As soon as visitors took one step into my mother's home on would go the kettle and the coffee table, well it was the 70s, would be filled with an array of sandwiches and cakes, but never was anyone ever asked the question, "Are you hungry?" Her mind had associated food with good hospitality, caring for her family and friends, along with the many other environmental cues that became part of her core belief system that is automatically enacted but never once questioned or challenged. The three-regimented-meals-a-day belief of my mother's was law. You could never miss a meal or you would go straight to prison and pay the price of my mother's strict judicial system. To see my mother upset or angry was something I never wanted to see, so I, as so many others still do, went through the motions. I became numb to the pain of overeating; that is, eating without hunger being felt. This caused the original and authentic programme, the Master Programme, to be overridden. A habit is the repetition of an action. Once accepted, the action is never again questioned or challenged, just performed. Seventeen percent of our day consists of conscious intent behaviours, or making a conscious decision to perform a specific action. That leaves a massive 83% of our actions left to unconscious learnt behaviours or habitual auto-behaviours linked to corresponding triggered associations. These are acted out unconsciously without any intelligent analytical conscious intervention attached. So if our learnt behaviours or habitual auto-behaviours are, in part, fallacious, then 83% of our daily behaviours are fallacious actions that contradict the original primal programme, or the Master Programme.

The difference between my mother and my grandfather was that my mother's original primal programme was changed and modified. She learnt to eat for reasons other than hunger, whereas my grandfather ate only when hungry. For him, stopping when satisfied was as natural as breathing. The results of these two very differently programmed people all point to a single and inevitable conclusion. My grandfather, living by his original unmodified programme, lived to be the ripe old age of ninety-one. He spent the last four days of his life in hospital, the first and last visit he ever made, and there he died peacefully. Up until then he had not visited a hospital or a doctor's surgery and no medical documentation could be attached to him. At ninety, he could walk briskly and still touch his toes. In fact his life changed very little between the ages of sixty to ninety, his mind and body functioning perfectly well. He never swallowed a tablet and was always planning tomorrow. If my grandmother hadn't passed away two years prior, then I think he could have easily been the man who lived forever. Now my mother, once again, a very different story. She struggles to walk; she has dedicated one cupboard to medication, and I am sure at times she can't bear to think about tomorrow because of the continuous pain she endures. So was my grandfather a very remarkable superhuman, one of a kind, or was it just that he followed nature's laws and my mother broke every one? And the conclusion, obesity is man's nemesis, the spoiler of life.

After observing these two people I soon became aware that learnt behaviours or habitual auto-behaviours (the formation of habit) and corresponding triggered associations based on a fallacious core belief system (limiting beliefs) are the true cause of human obesity. It is not specific foods that make us overweight but the behavioural manner in which these foods are eaten. The fundamental reason why conventional restrictive diets don't work. We, each and everyone of us, are all born with inherited instincts as part of the original primal programme to live a life of perfect health, but I saw that we are all continuously being reprogrammed by the world in which we live. This reprogramming modifies and changes the Master Programme, and soon is accepted as fact by the unconscious mind, the programme within the computer, which forms a new and unreliable fallacious core belief system. The most long-term and damaging reprogramming inflicted at an early age is the pattern of insisting upon three regimented meals a day passed on from one generation to the next. This is without doubt one of, if not the, most significant learnt behaviours or habitual auto-behaviours that attributes to obesity by forming the limiting belief that such behaviours are needed for survival. Eventually the unconscious mind begins to respond to the data of the new programme. No one can be blamed because the programmer, the parent, guardian or other authoritarians in a child's infancy, believes that what they are doing is for the child's best interest. Yet this is due to their own learnt behaviours or habitual auto-behaviours. They just pass on the make up of their own distorted, unreliable and fallacious core belief system; this cycle has to be broken. I noticed that we never see an obese wild animal or wild animals in need of constant medical attention. I knew that the cause of human and indeed domestic pet's early demise and ill health must be something unnatural. It didn't take me long to notice that we never see a wild animal eating and drinking in the main anything other than what they were originally designed to eat and drink: their primal foods. We humans have lost our original natural inherited instinctive eating programme. It's become distorted, unreliable, modified and changed due to environmental cues and fallacious beliefs. We are no longer living a natural instinctive life as we were first adapted to live. Our lives are constantly being modified, changed and reprogrammed by external forces, which become accepted as fact as new and contrived learnt behaviours, auto-behaviours, associations and spurious limiting beliefs become embedded. The programme we started our life with is now unrecognisable and unreadable by the human computer. We are following a rogue programme that is not one hundred percent compatible with the original primal blueprint of human existence – we have lost natural instinctive eating. The only way we will ever stop the obesity epidemic that is rapidly sweeping through the world is by educating expectant parents so that our future children will live their lives according to their original primal programme, the Master Programme, and not allowing it to be rewritten by authors ill-qualified.

A good analogy of the programme within the computer is to imagine the brain (tangible organic matter) as the computer and the mind within the brain as the programme (intangible). Once the unconscious mind, the programme, accepts something as fact, it will believe this fact to be true 100% of the time. Something repeated over and over again soon and easily becomes a new learnt behaviour or habitual auto-behaviour, and forms corresponding triggered associations, after which no conscious thought or intervention is needed to produce the actionable behaviour. But fear not, unconscious learnt behaviours or habitual auto-behaviours and all their triggered associations can easily be changed. By consciously recognising (self-insight) and challenging these habitual behaviours we can easily reset and reprogramme the unconscious mind to recalibrate to the authentic Master Programme of natural instinctive eating, that is eating for hunger and not environmental cues, responding only to the body's natural hunger and satiety signals, thus strengthening the signals within the cybernetic loop – the mind-body connection. The systematic method most successful to reignite natural instinctive eating is, *Acknowledge, Reprogramme, Succeed* as part of *Talk Yourself Slim With The Self-Chatter Diet.*

To reignite natural instinctive eating you have to first **Acknowledge** – ask your inner voice am I hungry or is it something else? Secondly, **Reprogramme** – by responding accordingly to the inner voice's answer; and thirdly **Succeed** – the conscious action will change the unconscious programme.

Your belief system will be the dominant factor and strongly influence the outcome and degree of your success. How much a person believes that they can lose weight is the golden key to *weight-loss success* along with the unshakeable desire to change. We have come to believe that losing weight is difficult due to the many failed diets. Each and every failure compounds the suggestion further. An internal locus of control is that we, each and everyone of us, takes full responsibility for our own actions, behaviours, outcomes and successes, creating the understanding that no one else can or will do it for us. We must take full control over our cognition, that is the way in which we process our thoughts into knowledge, as this in turn will give us domination over our own life, emotions and thinking. You have to believe one hundred percent that you can. As my grandfather would say, "If you know you can you will, if you know you can't you won't."

Emotional eating is also, mainly, nothing more than learnt behaviours or habitual auto-behaviours that responds to corresponding triggered associations produced from fallacious beliefs. An actionable habitual behavioural belief acts as a distraction from an upsetting or out-of-control situation, past or present, but more often than not recent. Emotional eating has become the world's greatest excuse for obesity, along with the fallacious and limiting belief that losing weight is difficult. Emotional eating is very counterproductive because it make two problems from the one. By eating to distract away from the original problem we actually create another by eating and then worrying about the perceived weight gain. People believe that eating a bar of chocolate will make them feel good or chocolate equals happiness, but they give no thought to the long-term effects of their actions. Once again by *Acknowledge, Reprogramme, Succeed* actionable habitual behavioural beliefs can easily be changed. The original primal programme, the Master Programme, of eating when hungry and stopping when satisfied, though dormant in some, can be reignited in all, as it forms the elemental composition of the human blueprint. For whatever reasons we have stopped listening, following and responding to our original programme can be overcome; it can, I assure you, be successfully and easily retrieved. When we listen and follow the original primal programme of natural instinctive eating, the body will easily achieve and maintain its own individual pre-set blueprint weight as decided on by nature at the time of individual human formation with the body then functioning efficiently and effectively, natural equilibrium is restored. Not storing food because of eating when food is not needed and also not storing food because of food restriction due to out-of-date conventional restrictive diets causes the body to trigger the famine mode, which, at all costs, it has to be kept out of to achieve and maintain *weight-loss success*. The human body is designed and programmed to survive and it will respond and react to the immediate environment whether natural or not. It is in all human interest to revert back to natural instinctive eating and follow the Master Programme. With the desire to change anything can be achieved, but there is no magic pill, no miracle cure and it is all down to you! Accept this and your battle is half won. Your body, more than anything else, wants to achieve and maintain its primal blueprint pre-set weight and there is only one person keeping it from *weight-loss success* and I think you know who that person is, don't you?

Talk Yourself Slim With The Self-Chatter Diet has evolved, developed and adapted from The Feelbetterfast Clinics original Inner-Voice Therapy and is inspired by my grandfather J. Arthur Laundon. The most critical person in your life is you! And it's the way in which you vocalise internally (self-chatter) that produces your outcomes, which is why you feel and act the distinctive way you do, even if you would otherwise prefer not to. We can, very easily, reprogramme the unconscious mind by simply changing the way in which we think, thus taking cognition control. Using the language of our inner voice in a more beneficially constructive and proactive way, we can evoke change by challenging our learnt behaviours or habitual auto-behaviours, disabling the destructive corresponding triggered associations, updating our fallacious core belief system by supplying more reliable information to reignite natural instinctive eating, and steadfastly follow the Master Programme. This is the principal of, *Talk Yourself Slim With The Self-Chatter Diet,* an efficacious psychological reprogramming technique to facilitate permanent weight loss. By forming an internal locus of control, you will be responsible for your own actions, behaviours, outcomes and successes, and not external forces. You will then, and only then, take control of your own life's destiny and achieve *weight-loss success!* Cognition control can only be taken by conscious intent, keeping a conscious awareness (mindfulness) of our thoughts and thinking until the new pattern of behaviour is formed and becomes accepted, normalised and habitualised by the unconscious mind, this is the fundamental aim of *Talk Yourself Slim With The Self-Chatter Diet.*

TALK YOURSELF SLIM WITH THE SELF-CHATTER DIET
COME ON, GIVE YOURSELF A GOOD TALKING TO!

I became totally obsessed with wanting to help people live an obese free life, and could not for the life of me see why others couldn't also see the obvious answer to obesity. It's not food that is the primary cause of obesity but the behavioural manner in which that food is eaten. Obesity is a chronic behavioural condition that unless addressed as such will continue to grow. With my burning ambition of saving the world from obesity through the changing of behaviours I trained as an holistic hypnotherapist with the National Association of Holistic Hypnotherapists (NAHH) with its teachings firmly based on analytical hypnotherapy – the foundations of a hypnotherapy practice. Later I achieved the level of Master Hypnotist with the British Academy Of Hypnosis (B.A.Hyp). My training as an hypnotherapist gave me a greater understanding of the conscious and unconscious mind concept, and how learnt behaviours or habitual auto-behaviours with all of their corresponding triggered associations and a fallacious core belief system can either make or break the quality of human life.

I am the founder of The Feelbetterfast Clinic, and also The National Behavioural Weight-Loss Programme. I am a pioneering leading authority on The Hypno-Gastric Band Procedure (The Original Dr Rockets™ Hypno-Gastric Band Procedure), promoting its use in behavioural change to facilitate permanent weight loss. Here I amalgamate all my knowledge, skills and findings to create the *Talk Yourself Slim With The Self-Chatter Diet,* so I can help people live an obese-free life, my obsession rewarded.

In this book you will discover all the secrets that throughout my life and work I have uncovered. Now within these pages I can reveal to the reader the true cause of obesity and offer a simple yet effective systematic method to solve the world's biggest disabler of human existence. Before you can apply a method you have to have a logical understanding of the mechanisms of the method being applied. You can then, and only then, apply the tools of the method to facilitate the changes to gain a successful and favourable outcome. I will remove all the myths put in place by the insidious diet industry to make weight loss appear difficult to form reliance on their unsustainable systems.

The definition of insanity is doing the same thing over

and over again and expecting different results. Now I am not implying in any way that habitual yo-yo dieters are insane, but it does make you think! All you need as the solution-seeker is the desire to change and to take full responsibility for your own actions, behaviours, outcomes and successes, in accordance with your health and well-being. Your weight affects no one other than yourself; it's an unnatural, abnormal obstacle that you have put in the way of your own health and happiness. Now is the time for its removal, bringing to a much timely end the Weight War, to finish a battle that should have never begun.

> *'The significant problems one has cannot be solved at the same level of thinking with which we have created them.'*

> Albert Einstein

Until obesity is accurately diagnosed and becomes generally accepted as a behavioural condition, and therefore treated as such, no solution will ever be found. From this book you can take as much or as little as you need to make all the changes necessary, to bring to a conclusion your own personal Weight War. Recognising (self-insight) your learnt behaviours or habitual auto-behaviours and triggered associations at a conscious level and then using the inner voice of self-chatter to intellectually analyse these habitual actionable behaviours, and respond accordingly with the appropriate action, your core belief system can easily be changed to return the human computer to its original settings and reignite natural instinctive eating, the genuine authentic programme written at the beginning of time by the original designer – the Master Programme. This book will also help people to recognise their behaviours and take action before the roots of obesity take hold, as prevention is better than cure. *Talk Yourself Slim With The Self-Chatter Diet* is a dieting revolution to *weight-loss success!*

JOHN RICHARDSON
'IT'S NOT MAGIC OR A MIRACLE, BUT IT DOES COME CLOSE.'

This book has fewer pages than the works of the great masters I admit, nor is it written in the same manner as a Dickensian novel or with grammar that Emily Brontë would be proud of. It is written to facilitate permanent *weight-loss success* and nothing more. If at times these words do appear repetitive, I assure you, it is by intent, as when each word of this book has been digested in a diligent manner, this repetition will have served its intended purpose.

NOW READ ON AND FIND ALL THE ANSWERS TO WEIGHT-LOSS SUCCESS...

CHAPTER ONE

INNER-VOICE THERAPY AND THE SELF-CHATTER DIET

*'The voice inside your head can be your best friend or
your worst enemy, your biggest critic or your No.1 fan.'*

J. A Laundon, 1909-2000

This book is not written with medical terms that the reader is unable to understand or makes the author appear Eton educated, nor will the reader be able to perform a surgical procedure at the end of reading it, due to the vast amounts of information provided on human biology. What can be guaranteed is that the reader will understand the general maintenance manual for the efficient and effective running of the body, the human machine. I don't have an in-depth knowledge of the workings of my car, but I do know that if I provide it with the correct fuel, water and oil, my car will function perfectly. The human machine is no different. If the human body is provided with the correct resources and it follows the original handbook, as written by the original designer, then the human body will function perfectly, with little or no problems occurring. If breakdowns do occur, it's usually down to operator error. The 'spanner in the works' is usually unnatural abnormal obstacles, of which one is obesity. The human body does have its own unique primal pre-set weight which the body continuously endeavours to maintain. In today's modern world that pre-set weight mostly fails amid all the unnatural fabricated obstacles we, ourselves, put in its path. Before we can achieve any degree of weight loss we have to remove these obstacles, thus clearing the way to *weight-loss success!* The aim of this book is to achieve a general understanding of the owner's manual for the trouble-free running of the body, the human machine.

Talk Yourself Slim With The Self-Chatter Diet is a systematic method combining conscious logical and informed communication along with unconscious psychological reprogramming techniques to achieve the desired objective of reigniting natural instinctive eating, following the Master Programme, facilitating permanent weight loss.

Every child that has ever been born, or indeed will ever be born, starts life with a clean slate, apart from the basic fundamental pre-written instincts hard-wired into the human computer that forms the Master Programme, which have the sole aim of survival and continuation of the human species. It is what we as adults write on this slate that will, over time, have a greater or lesser effect on the core belief system of each individual child, thus creating human individuality. As adults we are all authors of our future generations and it is of vital importance that we remain at all times conscientious, taking care to dot all the i's and cross all the t's. We cannot write in a fictitious fantasy style; we must be factual and always remember the importance of the task, especially as careless, shoddy work will reflect within the end product. We are all without doubt, and to many and varying degrees, reprogrammed with incorrect information, which leads to the formation of limiting beliefs or a fallacious core belief system that stops us from reaching our full potential and achieving success within our lives. The most damaging limiting belief and the one that has the most detrimental impact on the quality of human life is the belief that we must eat three regimented meals a day: breakfast, dinner and tea (food dictation). This is the rogue programme that, in the main, leads to obesity. The majority of incorrect and distorted information that is the catalyst for the formation of these limiting beliefs is received while still a child, usually in the first twelve years of life. This is before the critical faculty of the mind is fully able to analyse each individual situation correctly, as until then a child interprets each message literally. A habit is the repetition of an action. Repeating any action over and over again will allow it in time to become a learnt behaviour or a habitual auto-behaviour with corresponding triggered associations. This means repeating the limiting belief of needing breakfast, dinner and tea causes the new formed learnt behaviour or habitual auto-behaviour with corresponding triggered associations to be built on incorrect and inaccurate information. The unconscious mind forms habits to keep the analytical conscious mind as free as possible to deal with unprecedented, not previously experienced or rarely occurring situations. The conscious mind can only deal with one thought at a time. For example, if I was telling you a story and someone else started telling you a more interesting story simultaneously, your conscious mind would be attracted to the more interesting story, flitting back and forth feeling obliged to listen to the first but fully concentrating on neither. Habits are the unconscious mind's way of turning routine actions into new learnt behaviours or habitual auto-behaviours, creating corresponding triggered associations that are acted out with no conscious intervention being attached as a consequence and this it does very well, at times too well. The unconscious can just as easily form a bad habit (non-beneficial) as it can form a good habit (beneficial); that is, if the information received by the unconscious mind is distorted, erroneous or inaccurate, the habitual auto-behaviour will be based on unreliable and incorrect information. Once the information received has passed the critical faculty of the mind, the unconscious mind will never again consider the stored information as anything other than fact. It will only act and respond according to the stored information, which now becomes part of that person's core belief system, but never again questioned or challenged. No future concern is shown, as to whether the habit is beneficial or non-beneficial to the individual affected. So the problem lies in that the unconscious mind is very clever but non-intellectual, so it does not analyse each and every situation individually but only relies on past stored knowledge or memories to compare with the present situation to produce an outcome. So if a habitual auto-behaviour is formed on the repetition of a limiting belief based on fallacious origins, then the habit will normally be non-beneficial to that person's life. The younger the child is, the fewer past experiences they have stored to compare to, so there is a greater chance of a distorted, unreliable and incorrect belief becoming solidified.

A limiting belief is a belief formed and stored within the unconscious mind that is believed to be true but causes detrimental effects to the quality of human life due to the fact that the belief has been formed on unreliable, distorted or incorrect information. The unconscious mind now relentlessly responds to this belief as fact, even though consciously with time the person knows these facts to be untrue.

The unconscious mind 'dominantly' wins when the two sides of the mind enter conflict when dealing with a situation. A limiting belief will override common logic to produce an unfavourable outcome even when there is conscious present evidence that the stored information is detrimental and incorrect. Nonetheless, this will bear no consideration when producing the final outcome.

A learnt behaviour, or habitual auto-behaviour with corresponding triggered associations is formed through the constant repetition of an action which is then attaching triggered responses. For example, a person will form the learnt behaviour or habitual auto-behaviour of having breakfast every morning whether they are hungry or not. By constantly repeating the action of eating breakfast every morning before leaving the house based on the belief that 'I can't leave the house without breakfast' the action soon becomes automatic. The triggered response occurs at seven thirty, breakfast will be eaten at 7.30am every morning with no conscious intervention being attached to the outcome of the produced action been performed.

The real danger is when you add limiting beliefs and learnt behaviours or habitual auto-behaviours and all their corresponding triggered associations together. The only possible outcome is *disaster!* So with a limiting belief that food equals happiness will form the auto-behaviour and responding triggered association of eating food when unhappy. There forms the foundations of emotional eating with no conscious intervention attached, responded to and never again questioned or challenged, we now have a limiting belief producing catastrophic effects on human life.

So we have now ascertained that the unconscious mind is our programme, clever but possessing little, if any, actual intelligence, it just works relentlessly to its programme in an uncompromising fashion. It is wholly animalistic and habit forming by nature with an unshakeable precedence for survival. And that the conscious mind is the source of our intelligence, analysing present situations in accordance to past stored information (knowledge), or memory. This is why in infancy there exists little if any stored information (knowledge) of any benefit to assist the conscious mind, which is why limiting beliefs are formed more easily. The unconscious mind possesses no concept of time, so information received and stored in early childhood forms the foundations of a belief system still as real and active today, as an adult, as it was when first formed as a child. If that information hurts us in any way the unconscious mind will repress that memory. This is when *Natural Analysis Hypnotherapy, the foundations of a hypnotherapy practice,* is needed to treat the underlying cause of presenting symptoms. So as you can see our core belief system is at the centre of all our life's successes and failures and that the changing of our beliefs is of paramount importance when dealing with *weight-loss success* or failure. As we grow, our intelligence forms a better understanding of the world in which we live, and we become more knowledgeable with a lesser chance of limiting beliefs forming unconsciously exists. I do hope this demonstrates the fundamental importance of how in a child's life the transference of knowledge and the accuracy of its delivery is truly in proportion to the suffering it can unintentionally cause.

'Our perceptions grow from the seeds of belief.'

The inner voice of self-chatter has become one of the most efficient and effective ways of changing limiting beliefs, learnt behaviours or habitual auto-behaviours, deactivating and neutralising corresponding triggered associations and facilitating a successful outcome to many problematic conditions. The voice inside your head can be your best friend or your worst enemy, your biggest critic or your No.1 fan. It's how we talk to ourselves that can change our behaviours and beliefs, by changing the way in which we internally talk (self-chatter) we can raise self-esteem, lower social anxiety, reduce fear, become free from phobias, panic attacks and obsessive-compulsive disorders (OCD). With the possibilities being endless, there is no limit to the success we can achieve and all by changing the way in which we talk to ourselves or simply by utilising the inner voice of self-chatter. When we use self-chatter in association with weight loss we use the inner voice to change the detrimental behaviours and beliefs that lead to obesity by internally vocalising and keeping mindful (self-insight) of these behaviours and beliefs that keep us from *weight-loss success.* Through the repetition of actions, born of a logical understanding, we form new beneficially constructive and proactive behaviours, consequently changing the limiting belief system from fiction to fact, fantasy to reality, deleting the old out-of-date virus riddled software and uploading new data into the human computer to receive a beneficial response. The inner voice of self-chatter stimulates the imagination, remember that imagination is the language of the unconscious mind and that, what we imagine, the unconscious mind endeavours to make our reality. An athlete should have won the race before the starting pistol is fired, and you should see yourself as how you want to be and not how you are, how you don't want to be – think as a thin person thinks. We can all be anything we want to be, fat or thin, a success or a failure, and it's how we think that makes us the individuals we are today. We have to form an internal locus of control, that means it's you, and you alone that's responsible for your own actions, behaviours, outcomes and successes, not an external locus of control, relying on external forces to create your success. The inner voice of self-chatter helps keep you mindful of your beliefs, behaviours and associations, facilitating the transition from detrimental limiting beliefs to current beneficially constructive and proactive beliefs, creating behaviours and associations to aid in the re-igniting of natural instinctive eating. This strengthens the signals within the cybernetic loop, so that the mind and body connect, and the body's intelligence is then allowed to achieve its natural pre-set weight, decided by nature, recalibrated by man. The human body functions best on instinct and intuition in accordance with its design. We have lost the origins of man simply by not following the Master Programme, only by returning back to instinctive, intuitive living and following the authentic Master Programme will the longevity of the species ever be guaranteed.

So to simplify, the only way to achieve *weight-loss success* is for you to become consciously aware (self-insight and self realisation), recognising your own limiting beliefs in order to reprogramme learnt behaviours, habitual auto-behaviours and their corresponding associations that triggers the action of eating, as these form the fundamental and radical cause of the contributing factors of clinical obesity. By using the inner voice of self-chatter we create a conscious mindful awareness that responds to the body's internal hunger and satiety signals. Using conscious wisdom and the analytical intelligence of the critical faculty of the human mind, the individual can create a new and logical understanding, responding with constructive and proactive beneficial actions. Through the repetition of these actions and through responding to the signals of the cybernetic loop that creates the mind-body connection, we can return the unconscious mind back to reading, responding and reacting to the authentic primal blueprint programming of natural instinctive eating and in doing so we can delete the rogue programme that is the mainstay of the world's obesity epidemic with the added effect of potentially eradicating the cause of early human demise. With the new behaviours created by intent and becoming normalised by the unconscious mind, new habits are formed reigniting natural instinctive eating reverting back to the Master Programme.

'Take cognition control to achieve weight-loss success!'

Talk Yourself Slim with the Self-Chatter Diet is a

systematic method evolved, developed and adapted from The Feelbetterfast Clinics Inner-Voice Therapy to change beliefs, behaviours and associations, reignite natural instinctive eating and thus facilitate permanent weight loss. Food does not make you fat per se, but the behavioural manner in which food is eaten does. Until weight loss is addressed by behaviour and treated as such, replacing out-of-date food based restrictive diets, then no solution will ever be found.

'The solution of every problem lies in understanding and applying a method'

J. Arthur Laundon, 1909-2000.

Before any method can achieve success, a clear and logical understanding of the method is of paramount importance, as without this the method is only 'pie in the sky' and no more different than most fad diets. *Talk Yourself Slim With The Self-Chatter Diet* is a systematic method divided into two modules. The first module follows a logical approach, giving a broad and in-depth understanding of why we become overweight, how we become overweight and how easily it is not to be overweight. The second module explains the instructive application of the method and its integration into everyday life. The two modules come together to achieve the one common objective *weight-loss success!*

Dr. Rocket's Talk Yourself Slim with the Self-Chatter Diet. 'Copied my many emulated by none!'

CHAPTER TWO

PREREQUISITE WORDS OF WARNING AND THE LOGICAL APPROACH: AN UNDERSTANDING OF THE SYSTEMATIC METHOD TO WEIGHT-LOSS SUCCESS

'No pain, no gain – weight-loss success.'

Before you the reader can achieve any degree of *weight-loss success* whatsoever, you must first and foremost have a steadfast desire to change, and be prepared to take full responsibility for your own actions and behaviours, as recognising this is the first rule of achieving *weight-loss success.* Everything in this world has a price and weight loss is no different. You will have to be prepared to pay the price for your own success, and the price is verging on extortion. It is your own actions and behaviours that has put your body into its present state of obesity and it has to be you and only you that has the desire to change and break free from this state. No one has ever eaten food by accident, no one has had a gun held to their head and been told, "Eat." You have through your own actions chosen to do so, which means you can also chose not to, providing adequate desire resides within yourself to stimulate the transformation. There is no room for laziness, idleness or blame transferrers, as in blaming other people for your failures. Obesity is no one else's fault but a person's own. This may seem harsh, but the truth really does hurt. There is no magic pill, no secret elixir, even the author of these works will not be able to give any guarantee or do it for you. The journey to achieving the body's natural ideal weight will be hard, and for some I regret to say too hard, but anything worth having is worth all the time and effort invested in achieving the desired outcome. You cannot be fooled and led into a false sense of easy success because it will take all the desire you possesses to achieve. Your determination will have to be almost tactile and you will have to hold onto it as thought it is your last breath, because without a change for some I hasten to say it probably will be. Desire is the single most vital ingredient in the strive for success. Without it nothing will be achieved in any field of choice. Weight loss systems, bariatric surgery (body modification without behavioural change), the Hypno-Gastric Band Procedure, or any number of the fad diets that proclaim permanent and instant weight loss to be easy are being very manipulative and fabricating the truth. They exploit the millions of desperate diet hunters tracking down the elusive trophy of their own natural ideal weight. Easy instant weight loss is a fantasy; a no-effort system has yet still to be found, though it probably never will be! The diet industry is a master of mind magic, creating an illusion that to many is believed true even though they know it's only a trick. The secret to achieving natural ideal weight is that you take full responsibility for your own actions, behaviours, outcomes and success, and have the desire to change. Forget the false promises the weight loss industry proclaim that they can guarantee you permanent and easy to achieve weight loss. They can't. It's a myth. The answer lies totally with you and the amount of desire you possess, and your acceptance of your responsibilities for your own free choices. Once this is understood, success will be yours. So the first step before any weight loss system can achieve any degree of success is to be 100% certain that desire resides within and that you, the solution-seeker, are ready to take full responsibility for achieving your own success. You must hold a firm belief in your own successful outcome with no room for movement. And the second is pride. If you have no pride in your own bodily appearance, will you have the pride and motivation to achieve the desired effect of *weight-loss success?* Animals maintain a high standard of bodily hygiene and pride, so cleanliness and an acceptable presentation of appearance must be part of the inherited genetics of all animals. If you have a couldn't-care-less attitude towards your own appearance, then it's nearly certain you will have a couldn't-care-less attitude towards your own body weight, affecting the degree of commitment to achieving the end result.

'The solution of every problem lies in understanding and applying a method.'

J. Arthur Laundon, 1909-2000

My grandfather J. A. Laundon passed on to me a priceless piece of advice which is vital to all life's successes. The solution of every problem lies in understanding and applying a method. These are true words of wisdom, because it is impossible to be successful at anything unless you understand the mechanism of the method you intend to apply, so to be successful takes a combination of knowledge and method. So first, the knowledge. This is the logical approach, an explanation to form an understanding of how we become overweight, why we become overweight and how easy it is not to be overweight. Followed by the method to apply, *Talk Yourself Slim With The Self Chatter Diet,* and you will achieve *weight-loss success!*

This is the part where I will revel to the reader all the secrets to achieving and maintaining their natural ideal weight in a logical and easy to understand format. These are the secrets the diet industry will never want you to know as they will end an era of antiquated restrictive dieting. And we all know that diets don't work, don't we? First, I ask you the reader, who is responsible for your weight management? The answer is hopefully obvious, but if not, your weight management is your responsibility and it will never affect one other person apart from yourself. It's inescapable, and without any doubt that the responsibility lies totally with you. Most people have what is known as an external locus of control; that is, they believe that external forces are responsible for the outcome and degree of success in all of their life's challenges and aspirations. They believe that the diet industry will solve all of their weight problems and they allow other people, circumstances and situations to control themselves. So forming an internal locus of control is another equally important factor in the achieving of *weight-loss success,* knowing

100% that **'YOU'** will be the one solely responsible for that successes, not someone or something else. By not allowing other people (external forces) to manipulate and control you, you will take back the controls of your own life's destiny, or in other words form an internal locus of control, not allowing other people, circumstances and situations to control you. It is up to you to make all the right choices. It is up to you to make the decisions. It is up to you to call all the shots. That is what an internal locus of control is: you are in control, producing your own successful outcomes. Do you actually think diet clubs are genuinely bothered or in the least bit concerned as to whether you lose weight or not? No! All they are concerned about is their weekly fiver! The time has come to turn your search inwards; take cognitive control, accept full responsibility for your own actions, behaviours, outcomes and successes, and thus create an internal locus of control, because you don't drive your car from the outside, do you?

	THE CONTROL OF DESTINY or THE LOCUS OF CONTROL	
I control my destiny (Internal)		Others control my destiny (External)

I ask you, the reader, do you have children? If your answer is yes, then I say only this to you: if you die for no other reason than being purely overweight, then of course at first your children will be sad, very sad, naturally. But they will get over it because life does go on with or without you. So in this scenario there is only one loser and that's you, because you literally have taken your own life and there is no one else to blame but yourself. Here's another question, do you think obesity should be accepted as a modern-day natural, normal state of being? I hope your answer here is no, but I do expect some to say yes with the explanation being that obese people are very nice, along with many other various and politically correct answers. But that wasn't the question I asked. I didn't ask whether they were nice people or not, of which I am sure many of them are. What I did ask was whether obesity should be accepted as a natural, normal state? And the answer is definitely not! It's not a natural normal state. It is a very unnatural, abnormal state. If we accepted obesity as a natural, normal state, then premature deaths would become even more premature, life expectancy would fall and the world would become an even more unhealthy place in which to live. So no: overweight, obese or dare I even say fat people should never be accepted as a normal state of being. People who proclaim that they are happy being overweight are the people I don't believe for one minute. How could they be? Obesity only makes life much more difficult than it needs to be, for no apparent beneficial reason. These are the same people who over time you will see keep trying to lose weight. Even the actress and comedian, who will, with all respect, remain unnamed, who has in numerous interviews proclaimed that she is very happy being the size she is, has been noted to have lost weight since finding a new partner. This proves the fact that obesity is an unnatural, abnormal state and not the preferred state to be in when bedroom antics return back into the equation.

Desire is the golden key to unlock the door of *weight-loss success*. Without desire you will achieve nothing, but with desire you can achieve anything. Equalled only by an internal locus of control formulating weight-loss success, therefore desire and an internal locus of control is the prerequisite of anything that you are aiming to be successful at. All this involves is you taking full responsibility for your own actions, behaviours, outcomes and success and not following environmentally fabricated prompts and cues. Here now is the explanation, or the logical approach, to gain an understanding of the systematic method of *Talk Yourself Slim With The Self-Chatter Diet.*

THE LOGICAL APPROACH

When you were a baby you cried when you were hungry, and you knew when you were satisfied; not allowing any more food into your mouth. If you didn't like the look, the taste or the smell of the food that you were being given, then you wouldn't eat it, mum usually ending up wearing it. So at this time in your life you had natural instinctive eating. As a baby your predictable daily modus operandi is: sleep, on waking cry, feed until satisfied and then return back to sleep. Your stomach was the perfect size for your body, not stretched and made oversized, out of shape due to eating for reasons other than hunger. So at this time in your life everything was perfect and just as it should be. You lived on instinct without any conscious intervention involved. You had, at this stage of life, natural instinctive eating, you simply ate when you were hungry and stopped when you were satisfied, just as nature intended. Then it all started to go wrong.

It all starts to go wrong with the very first plate of food you are ever given, for who gave you this food? That's right, your mother, parent or guardian. I call this parental intervention, or 'mother knows best' or 'so she thinks'. She, your mother, then starts to dictate (food dictation) to you when you will eat, what you will eat, the amount you will eat, and will even make noises like trains, lorries, boats and planes to try to force even more food into your stomach. She will call you in from play, telling you it's time to eat, even though a child will never starve – trust me they will always come home when they are hungry. She may just as well put a funnel into your mouth and pour your food in with you having no say in the matter whatsoever. She will use bribes, threats, treats and rewards. The threat could be if you don't eat all of your dinner, then you can't play out with your friends, or worse still, not allowing you to leave the table until you present an empty plate for mother's inspection, the treat, the reward, a lovely treacle sponge and custard. If you put a main course and a pudding in front of a child and say eat as much as you want then when you have finished off you go and play with your friends, the child will eat a small amount of one, then a small amount of the other, then off they'll go to play with their friends – no damage done. But parents don't allow this to happen. Parents say, "If you don't eat all of your main course then you cannot have a pudding." The pudding now becoming a desired object. So the child will eat half the first course, feel satisfied knowing that enough food has been eaten, but will suffer the pain of eating the other half even though they are not hungry, because they now see the pudding as a reward for eating all of the first course. And worse still is when parents bring emotions into the equation. They say, "Come on, eat all of your dinner for Mummy. Mummy will be very upset if you don't clean your plate and save me from the washing up" – membership accepted for the clean plate society, ker-ching! What child would want to see their mother upset? Or dad will say, "Come on, son, eat up all of your dinner or you won't grow up to be a big boy like Daddy." Once again, what small boy doesn't want to grow up to be a big boy like Daddy? Emotion is a very powerful reprogrammer! The child perceives the pudding as a reward for eating all of the main course, so the child then starts to eat to receive the reward and the praise. They are now eating for another reason other than hunger. The pudding now seen as a reward for eating all of their dinner and not simply just food for fuel any more. You must learn to see things as the literal child, not an analytical adult!

'Every child is born with a clean slate and it's what we as adults write on that child's slate that dictates what that child will become. We are the authors of that child's life, so always write with care to avoid future repair!'

J. A Laundon, 1909-2000.

Rewarding with food is no different than training a puppy to fetch a stick. Parents will say to a child, "If you can sit still and keep quiet for half an hour, if you can do that for Mummy, I will give you some chocolate, but only if you can complete the full thirty minutes, can you do that?" The laying of the gauntlet, but whose benefit is this game really for? No child will care about the chocolate, all they care about is proving to mum or dad that they can do this. So the child will sit perfectly still, arms crossed, bolt upright, not even blinking. After the thirty minutes is up the parent thinks that was fantastic because they got their thirty minutes of piece and quiet to have lunch and watch *Loose Women*. They will give the child a big hug and tell him/her how well he/she has done and then present the child with the chocolate, the prize, the reward. The child is now highly emotional, to the child it's like winning a gold medal at the London Olympics 2012 and the chocolate is stored in the unconscious mind as the source of a good feeling, pleasure; forming the basis for future, so called, emotional eating. The unconscious mind avoids pain and is naturally programmed to replace pain with pleasure. So when pain is felt whether emotional or physical, the mind will go through all its stored files trying to find the ones labelled good feeling. Bingo, chocolate, that will make you feel good. It was never the chocolate, it was the whole sequence of events leading to the chocolate that created the good feeling; but the non-analytical unconscious mind has forgot everything else and labelled the chocolate as the cause of the good feeling creating the association that food equals happiness: wrong! Once accepted by the unconscious mind it is never again questioned or challenged and has become a cue for blue-light rapid response. Hypothetically speaking, the puppy has retrieved the stick. Birthdays, Christmas and Easter all produce forms of food based associations, that is, associating food with the state of being happy. So the next time you are eating chocolate ask yourself this question, "Am I eating this chocolate for no other reason than hunger satiety, or is it something else?" Our behaviours are a low 17% conscious and a massive 83% unconscious or automatic, so we live the largest percentage of our lives on automatic response, actions and behaviours. This is why consciously we know what to do to lose and manage our weight, but when concentration or will power is relaxed we will return back to following the spurious unconscious programme with all it's auto-responses attached to associated situations. The problem is the unconscious mind has no concept of time. Things are now as they have always been and always will be. Unless reprogrammed by accident or intent, the clever but non-analytical unconscious mind will just relentlessly follow the modified programme unaware of the consequence of the produced action, maybe for the rest of the person's life, for example, associating chocolate with a good feeling. So if we go through an extended period of time being unhappy, we will add to our weight for what at first appears as no apparent reason, but by now the reason should be becoming more clear!

'A child will become what it's taught to become.'

J. A Laundon, 1909-2000

When we eat to cover emotions (emotional eating), it is only a temporary distraction from the original underlying problem. Food can certainly affect our minds, becoming an automatic response to stress and unhappiness. Emotional eating is very counterproductive and does nothing more than create further problems, because the problem you were eating to cover will still be there and now a new problem has been created, as you have just eaten a bar of chocolate the size of the kitchen table. The one problem has now become two, the original problem plus the perceived weight gain. If you feel emotional hunger then do something else, something enjoyable: take a walk, stroke the cat, paint a picture, read a book, in fact anything other than eat, because eating will after the event only make things twice as bad. To cease emotional eating you have to 1. *ACKNOWLEDGE* – ask your inner voice am I hungry or is it something else? 2. *REPROGRAMME* – respond appropriately to the inner voice's answer. 3. *SUCCEED* – the conscious action will change the unconscious programme. Remember, food does not make you happy, it actually has the reverse effect! The unconscious mind develops sophisticated defence mechanisms that reinforce our core beliefs with some being logical and beneficial but also some being illogical and non-beneficial. It's as though the unconscious mind has to prove its beliefs. By a process of self-insight, realising and recognising, these beliefs can be questioned, challenged and changed – **A**cknowledge, **R**eprogramme, **S**ucceed, *weight-loss success!*

Nostalgia; picture this scenario. It's Sunday afternoon and you are four years old. You are sitting with Grandma and Granddad all cosy on the sofa in front of a warm log fire watching your favourite film. Halfway through the film, Granddad brings out the chocolate, life could not get any better. Thirty years later you may be feeling pain whether emotional or physical; Grandma and Granddad may no longer be around, so what is left of this scenario?

Chocolate. Your mind will have associated chocolate with this memory and a good feeling. Everything is forgotten apart from the chocolate labelled good feeling, and once again, you've guessed it, when feeling down out comes the chocolate. It could also have labelled the film with good feeling, so when you feel down out comes the film you watched thirty years ago – now that's not too bad as films have far less calories than chocolate.

By using bribes, threats, treats and rewards, all we are doing is puppy training our children. Habits are formed through the continuous repetition of an action. By rewarding for eating, we are reprogramming the unconscious mind (17% conscious behaviours, 83% unconscious behaviours) and forming new falsified learnt behaviours or habitual auto-behaviours with corresponding triggered associations, which put obstacles in the path of success and modify the original primal programme of eating when hungry and stopping when satisfied. We have taught the unconcious mind, the programme within the brain, to override our natural hunger and satiety signals so they have no impact. We have to now restore and return hunger sensitivity to the intelligence of the body. From the day we are born until we are presented with our first plate of food, it is other people that take control of our eating habits. First, parents, teachers, then as we get older socialising peer pressure, then, when we become overweight, diets. A child will never starve, they may not eat as much as a parent thinks they should eat, but they will always eat the right amount of food they need to survive. A child is born with natural instinctive behaviours, it's adults that take that instinct away. So by force-feeding a child to eat food when he or she is not hungry, all you are doing is reprogramming their computer, their unconscious mind, to eat non-instinctively, to eat for reasons other than hunger. The original programme is being overridden, modified and changed – problems are now on the horizon. If we brought up a child in a more 'animalistic' way, by only providing primal foods and water so the child can feed freely on demand, I can guarantee you this, the child would remain slim and more importantly healthy. A newborn lamb is not told where to find milk, it instinctively knows. For some reason, we feel human offspring should eat the amount of food parents think they should eat and not the amount of food they themselves know they should eat instinctively. So we use bribes, treats, threats and rewards along with the many other tools in our force-feeding repertoire, intensively farming our children into a lifetime of obesity, taking the lamb to the slaughter – it's a crazy old world in which we now live.

'Parents should make food available, nothing else.'

J. A. Laundon, 1909-2000

Enforcing regimented breakfast, dinner and tea creates the rogue programme that in the main leads to obesity! Set meal regimes are at the root cause of most, if not all human obesity and early demise, because it stops the body's natural food/fuel regulatory/compensatory system working efficiently and effectively, or in other words implements food dictation. What moon-struck lunatic came up with this idea then? I ask you the reader, do you eat breakfast? If the answer is yes, then I will now ask you, are you hungry every morning at breakfast time? Usually the answer is sometimes, but not every time. So why do you have breakfast when you're not hungry? The reply is usually you just do, but this is probably because you were told as a child that breakfast is the best meal of the day, breaking the fast! Breaking the fast is the most ridiculous answer I have ever heard as you know you have been fed the day before and that you are not fasting, only sleeping. If you wake in the morning and you are not hungry then you have enough fuel on board at that precise moment in time. If you wake up in the morning and you're hungry, then you eat breakfast because fuel is running low and more fuel needs to be taken on board. Would you put fuel into your car every morning if the fuel tank was registering full? Thought not. All you are doing by mindlessly eating food when you're not hungry is filling your body's storerooms with lipids, because the food you are consuming is simply not needed. We become programmed by receiving and accepting false information as part of our core belief system and this is being passed on from one generation to the next with these beliefs never being questioned or challenged. No one will ever convince me that everyone in the whole wide world is hungry at precisely five o'clock everyday, it just can't happen. The majority of people who are overweight eat by the clock and not by how hungry they feel. In fact most people will not be able to remember the last time that they felt genuine hunger. Equalled only by sex, hunger is part of a system of self-preservation and one of our most powerful driving forces. When genuine hunger is felt, then the mind cannot concentrate on anything other than finding food, triggering the hunter gather mode. If, for example, someone says that when they are working they can distract their mind away from hunger, then this is not genuine hunger and food is most definitely not needed. What stops us all from reverting back to cannibalism is nothing more than cupboards full of food as when in times of extreme hunger we will revert to eating our own if that's what it takes to survive. But also remember the limiting belief of food makes you happy. If your job makes you unhappy, then the unconscious mind will try to make you happy by prompting you to eat for a reason other than hunger to distract away from the job you hate. We are told we shouldn't eat after 7pm, but why? If you are hungry, then you need food/fuel. You wouldn't let your car run out of fuel would you? Also guilt is another factor. If someone cooks a meal for you, then you feel unappreciative and guilty if you don't empty your plate, hungry or not. By doing this all you are doing is allowing someone else to control you, damaging your body, the most precious possession you have. A predominate problem is that we all accept but never question and challenge our beliefs especially when they have originated from an authoritarian source!

'If my name was Mr. Morning Breakfast Cereal and I told you that breakfast was the best meal of the day, would this be because I care about you or would it be to get my hands on your hard earned cash?'

If you read the recommended serving on a box of breakfast cereal biscuits it will always say two per serving, but how do they know how hungry you are? You accept their advice as fact, but is it fact or is it that if you only ate one then the box would last twice as long, which is not good for profit? Notice when the advertisements are shown for breakfast cereal biscuits on TV they never fail to show the actors eating two. TV is the most powerful subliminal form of reprogramming, whether true or false, to the unconscious mind. This is why some people think Coronation Street is a real place and write to the actors addressing the envelope to the character's name. So now lets imagine it's teatime and you are a little hungry, your evening meal is served up and you begin to eat. You are going to eat all of this meal because: 1. You've bought the food. 2. You or someone else has cooked the food. 3. Most importantly, it's teatime. You eat half the meal and you feel satisfied, but I know you are going to eat the other half of the meal for the reasons previously mentioned. The half you ate when you were hungry, that's fine because you will burn this amount of food as it was needed. The half you ate when you were satisfied (full), no longer hungry, you will store as fat. This perfectly designed and flawless natural survival system worked perfectly well thousands of years ago when you were sat in your cave and you became hungry. You then had to go out and either hunt for meat or gather fruit, vegetables, nuts, leaves, pulses, etc. This all took time and effort, so you would use your naturally stored fat to survive until you had hunted and gathered enough food to satisfy your hunger and refuel your body. Naturally stored fat does not look the same as abnormal fat. The fat you naturally store for survival does not hinder or hamper your health and fitness in any way and is not visible as the unnatural, abnormal fat is, you know, the fat that is now hanging over the top of your jeans. If people today had to hunt and gather their food to survive, obesity would not be at epidemic levels. I would dare to say it would not exist because the environment would naturally regulate and dictate human weight. Bear in mind, too, that if you ate a little too much food back in the times of our cavemen ancestors, this did not pose much of a problem because you never knew where your next meal was coming from, so natural food regulation/compensation naturally occurred. Do you ever see a fat fox? When Mr Fox wakes in the mornings, he can't say, "What are we having for breakfast, dear?" He will have to go out and make a kill, and he will not be successful every time, especially if he became overweight, so once again natural regulation/compensation of food/fuel occurs. What do you do when you are hungry? You get up, walk to a well stocked fridge, open the door and as if by magic, hey presto, food – a human intensive fattening system. How much effort did that take? And in fact, were you really hungry on decision to eat? Every time you eat when you're not hungry (those last dozen mouthfuls of every meal) you store an amount of fat, and you do it again, and again, and again. The human store cupboard becomes fuller and fuller, but when do you ever need to draw on this stored fat? Never! What makes you overweight is all the food you eat when you're not hungry, predominantly by the running of the rogue programme of three regimented meals a day, breakfast, dinner and tea (food dictation), along with other habitual auto-behaviours and associations that have been formed through false information being accepted as fact. Fortunately, or unfortunately, we now never have to endure times of food scarcity, but the question posed is which is worse – food scarcity or modern-day food abundance? Now that's a ponderer.

'The world in which we all live has evolved, the human body has not.'

We think we live in a modern world that is perfectly suited to sustain all human life, but this is a fallacy. The human body was designed to survive in the environment it was originally designed for and created to live in, as a hunter gatherer. The human is very robust and resilient and does not need wrapping up in cotton wool with everything being given on a plate – pardon the pun. It functions best without food dictation and routine set meals. Food scarcity instinctively triggers the hunter-gather mode of self-preservation which believe it or not resides within all of us. This has the added effect of producing motion to survive: exercise. Hunger is a human driving force, as when we are hungry nothing else will enter the mind but finding food and, as a consequence, spontaneously triggering the hunter gatherer mode; the ancient instinct to survive. However, this is a feeling I fear today very few ever feel. We are now living in a modified and fabricated world that would be unrecognisable to our former hunter-gatherer selves. We live in a world of unnatural, abnormal obstacles, with processed foods, alcohol and hidden sugars all contributing to the dominance of obesity. The greatest threat to mankind is profiteering food manufacturers who provide food for profit with no concern or consideration in production for the benefit of human health. People now overindulge, and become addicted to the sweet taste of processed/refined sugar (taste addiction) or suffer alcohol abuse. They say they want to lose weight, but they are not prepared to forsake these manufactured obstacles. The reason a cow, pig or sheep becomes fat is because it is kept in a restricted area, fed unlimited amounts of food; it is intensively farmed. If these animals were in their natural state then they would have to roam and search to find their food, and food would never be guaranteed. We are no different than farmed animals that are being intensively fattened for slaughter in what is now an unnatural environment for healthy human existence as was first originally intended. We think we are so privileged to live in a country where food is cheap, affordable and always available. We abuse this privilege instead of appreciating it. This abuse is driven by greed not survival. We see this greed all around us, especially emphasised when staying in hotels at morning breakfast. Because the breakfast is all-in, people will eat as much as they can so that they, as they see it, get their money's worth. But they will eat habitually again at dinnertime and again at teatime, storing more and more fat, and because we now never experience times of food scarcity the stored fat is never called upon in its intended form to ensure human survival. Humans hold more stored food than supermarkets after a delivery. In some parts of the country, obesity has now reached an all time high of 1 in 3. So forget the all-day breakfasts because they are just a brilliant sales ploy to increase profits. You know you will eat again that day! The body's natural food regulatory/compensatory system cannot work efficiently and effectively if you succumb to food dictation instead of instinctively eating when refuelling is actually needed.

> *'Peak performance is achieved with the designer's*
> *choice of fuel.'*

Your body is a human machine and your metabolism is your engine. Food enters the body through the mouth, goes down into the stomach and is metabolised into energy to drive the human machine, with the waste products then being evacuated. You do have your own fuel gauge, your hunger. When it's on **E** you're **E**mpty, you eat for energy; when it's on **F** you're **F**ull, STOP. This system works perfectly with problems only occurring when you don't listen and respond to this gauge, and eat when you're not hungry. When you make a conscious decision to eat food when the gauge is still showing full, food enters the stomach and the metabolism (your engine) says, "What is this person doing, fuel is not needed, this delivery was not ordered." Imagine your stomach as a factory and running the factory are a work force of hundreds of little workers feeding the metabolism, your engine, with food/fuel to power your body. On the side of your stomach is a great big bell. When food/fuel is needed the bell is rung, you will become hungry and food/fuel should always be delivered on time. But you don't wait for the bell to be rung, do you? You just keep delivering food/fuel and the workers end up saying, "We have nowhere to store this food, all the storerooms are full to capacity. We'll just have to force more in. Come on, lads, push." So the storerooms, your hips, around your middle, and the biggest one of all, your bum, are all bursting full, the walls bulging into all sorts of shapes, but the delivery has to go somewhere. To make matters even worse you don't wait till the bell is rung again before you pile in even more food/fuel. You can see what's going to happen, your workers are working in unacceptable conditions, there's going to be an industrial walkout and the factory will one day shut down! The more serious damage happens when the blood stream becomes full of unwanted and unneeded glucose. The natural production of insulin cannot deal with the copious amounts of glucose caused by eating when food is not needed. Also we are now more than ever eating more and more processed foods, all loaded to capacity with refined/processed sugar causing the natural balance of the human body to become disturbed and unbalanced. Microwave ready-meals made for convenience were not designed for the healthy running of the human body; they were mostly produced for the profits of the big food companies rather than the health of the nation. Tinned foods are full of hidden and secret sugars; foods we know are healthy are unhealthy in their processed form; and the biggest obstacle of all is alcohol. It has become a Weight War and the odds are stacked heavily against the human body winning. All of this unbalance and lack of the body receiving it's natural fuel (primal foods) is leading to the biggest problem within the health service, and demise in human health: diabetes. Blood pressure, hypertension (the silent killer), are others, because the body cannot continue carrying this unwanted and unnatural weight, it was never designed to. Thyroid dysfunction, chemical imbalances, adds to the mix. I believe that a high percentage of thyroid imbalance in patients are predominately caused by snacking, eating when not hungry. This causes a chemical imbalance within the human body. When you feel hunger, this triggers all the chemical reactions within the metabolism to prepare to receive and process food. When you eat for reasons other than hunger, then the chemical reactions are on standby and not expecting a delivery of food. Panic sets in and the system becomes out of balance, disharmony prevails as hunger is the trigger for the process to begin. The thyroid depends on iodine for its functioning, so the constant eating of processed foods can cause a deficiency. Iodine can be gained from eggs, shellfish, salt-water fish, seaweed; all helping to prevent thyroid dysfunction. Natural instinctive eating resolves numerous metabolic problems, rebalancing the body's natural equilibrium.

'Eat foods in their natural state to receive all the elements needed that sustain human life.'

Overweight people believe that if they could have the fat sliced from their stomach, hips and bottom, then everything would be OK, problem solved. But the real problem lies not on the outside of the body, but on the inside. On the inside of your body are located all your organs. Every organ in your body has to move freely, to work efficiently and effectively. Imagine if all your organs are surrounded in cold chip fat (visceral fat), how will this effect their performance? Yes, it's going to make it twice as hard for them to function and eventually in time this could be the cause of them ceasing to function altogether. It's not generally understood that obesity is not only subcutaneous (external under the skin fat, the fat we care about, vanity fat) fat but also visceral (internal) fat. More people are now producing visceral fat, looking externally acceptable but internally obese causing organ restriction and premature death. A high percentage, probably 75%, of all doctor's and hospital appointments are caused through stress or obesity. Stress and obesity are the underlying cause of most of the presenting symptoms we visit our doctors with. Common sense says that if I am overweight then simply by removing the obstacle of obesity I will achieve perfect health, and that is exactly what you will do. You haven't broken anything, all you have done it put a great big boulder in the way of your natural healing system. By the simple removing of that boulder then your stomach will retract, the size of your hips and bum will reduce, and all your organs will move freely again and perfect health will be yours, natural equilibrium restored. Fat is an essential component within the human body, it only becomes a problem when in excess. Excess fat is the direct result of our actions at one time or another!

'We expect nothing less from a diet than mass weight loss when in fact weight-loss success is slow and subtle.'

The reason why diets don't work is that they were never meant to, now there's a surprise, right? Diets equal profit! If diets worked then there would only need to be the one, and there are always thousands in print at any one time, need I say more?

> *'The definition of insanity is doing the same thing over and over again expecting a different result!'*

So these are the true facts – If today you visited your doctor with weight issues, more likely than not he would give you a NHS diet sheet or put you on a weight loss programme. But how would he or the NHS know what your daily actions would be in accordance with your calorific requirement for that specific day – unless he was a soothsayer. The diet sheet would say that a woman needs 2,000 calories per day (approx.) to function and a man 2,500 (approx.) but it does not tell you that you do not need the same amount every day because each day of your life is variable. If you are having a sofa Sunday then you will not need as many calories as you would on a day when you're running a marathon, or even when you go on a shopping spree to Meadowhall (not sure between Meadowhall and a marathon which you would need the most calories for?) So let's say today is a day when your body needs 2,000 calories. If you give it 1,000 like some restrictive diets or even 400 like the more severe shake and bar diets, then your body is not receiving enough calories to function and regenerate itself with the body then entering famine mode causing fat to store. If you go above the 2,000 calories needed, then once again you will only store fat because overeating is a deliberate preparation for a famine with the extra food being converted to lipids – stored energy. I agree, at this moment it looks like a no-win situation, but bear with me.

Now let's see how the diet clubs operate. First, when you enrol at your favourite diet club, why don't you ask to see the proof of their product or system over the last five years? Would you buy another product without first knowing the product worked and how good that product was? I would be very doubtful that they could show you any proof, because diets don't work, do they? They have promised you something that they can very rarely deliver. Also because it's only a small amount of money invested each week if it does fail does it really matter anyway? But five pounds a week over a twenty-five-year period adds up to be a hell of a lot of cash and a lot of wasted time and effort just to be crowned a yo-yo dieter. One of my clients worked with a lady who lost eleven stones with a well-known diet club, she became slimmer of the year. Within months after achieving her goal weight she was well on her way to putting all the weight back on. The diet clubs used her picture for years after she had put every last pound of the weight back on, and a little more. Another client came to see me and said that she knew diets didn't work because she had attended a diet club in her own village. The lady who was leading the group was stood between two large photographs of herself before and after the weight loss. This client for her own reasons decided not to carry on attending the diet club. Six months later she saw the same group leader coming out of Marks & Spencer's and, in her own words, she was the same size as the back end of a double-decker bus. The conclusion she came to was that if it didn't work for the diet club leaders then how could it have possibly worked for her? Also, she said, they change their systems as often as she changed her underwear. So what does that tell you? Any diet that restricts the body of the food it needs when hungry will fail! OK, so you decide to join a slimming club and the predictable course of your attendance is this. The first part you do really well because: 1. You have paid your £5. 2. You are focused, it's a new adventure! 3. Fear, fear that you don't want to be the only woman/man who doesn't lose weight (don't eat till after the weigh-in, wear light cloths with empty pockets, have a wee first, who are you fooling?). 4. When you lose weight by a restrictive diet you will lose more muscle than fat. The diet clubs know this and want this to happen because muscle weighs more than fat, so this shows a false weight loss but compounds the diets club's suggestions that their systems are working. 5. Your mind has not twigged onto the fact that you are starving your body of the food that it actually needs.

In the second part you obviously and inevitability fail. Usually the failure will be attributed to eating a tiny piece of cake, or some other 'sin' food. In a piece of cake there will be approximately 200 calories. You need 3,500 calories (approx) over your daily intake to put one pound of weight on, so the one piece of cake now looks very insignificant. What has happened is that your mind has learnt that if you have one piece of cake then you will say, that's blown the diet, I'll start again on Monday, even though its still only Tuesday, and you will eat twenty-seven more pieces of the cake. When you become hungry and your body needs food, the mind's natural survival instincts jump into action (the mind sees restriction of food as a threat to human life) and will find a way of getting the food that's needed for human existence – the master survivor. Forget Ray Mears and Bear Grylls, they are amateur in comparison! You have broken your diet so many times in this predicable and habitual fashion that it has become a learnt and limiting behaviour, so your mind sabotages your diet to receive the food/fuel actually needed to sustain life. Then what happens is, after your attendance ceases, the diet club contacts you and says, we are missing you, come back and join us and take advantage of our, be a fool to miss, free rejoining offer. So you think to yourself, well I did do well at the beginning, and this is exactly what they want you to think; everything going to their plan. So you start the process all over again and earn yourself the undistinguished title of yo-yo dieter. Yo-yo dieting makes you fat and feel a failure! Most, if not all diets rely heavily on food restriction, along with fear and shame, to suggest to their many loyal and devout followers that their unsustainable systems are having the desired effect of *weight-loss success:* the true reason for the weekly weigh-in. This usually only being short lived, and at times even causing food deprivation, with the body then responding with retaliation and as a consequence of nature producing further weight gain. Tests were concluded and published as far back as the 1950s (Ancel Keys, The Biology Of Human Starvation), in which people were starved then fed unlimited amounts of food. The concluding results showed that when food was restricted then made unrestricted, many people ate in the region of eight times more food over the following twelve week period, once the restriction had been lifted. This accounts for why people on a restrictive diet lose half a stone then put three quarters of a stone back on. So all conventional orthodox restrictive diets do is make you fat and feel a failure. With the failure of each new diet tried you feel that you are being pushed further and further into a corner with nowhere else to go with the solution becoming even more elusive. The conclusion is that diet clubs using out-of-date restrictive dieting methods should really be called *fat clubs*, why? Because they make you fat and feel a failure, FACT! As far back as 1950 it was proven that conventional restrictive diets don't work, and if they did then there would only need to be the one. Food based restrictive diets or in fact any diet that involves calorie counting restrictive methods are the work of charlatans, offering false hope to their loyal minions; because the failure is not your fault, its inevitable!

'It only hurts when you want it so bad.'

People will blame glands, thyroid, water retention, medication, giving all sorts of excuses for being overweight, but think about this: how do you fatten a pig? You feed it. If you don't feed it then it won't grow.

By keeping a pig in a restrictive, unnatural environment with an unnatural, constant supply of food the pig will respond in an equally unnatural way and become fat. People are constantly searching for the magic pill to *weight-loss success,* taking one pill and when that pill fails taking a different one. I had a bariatric surgeon attend *The Feelbetterfast Clinic* for *The Lose Weight And Feel-Better-Fast System Of Natural Weight Management,* incorporated within the system, *The Hypno-Gastric Band Procedure,* and she told me that she had just recently done one of the well-known shake-and-bar diets where a large water intake is part of the programme. I asked her how, with all her medical knowledge, she could even think it could or would work? She said, "When you're desperate, darling, you will try almost anything because you think it may just work for you." So even people who are specialists in the medical world will hope that they too find the magic formula to *weight-loss success,* and the truth is regrettably there isn't one! If you wonder why people like Victoria Beckham, Rosemary Conley and top catwalk models all stay so thin, it is because their careers depend on it, fear! A naturally thin person eats when hungry and stops when satisfied, eating for no other reason other than hunger. The human body has a primal blueprint weight – a pre-set weight. If you go above your pre-set weight then the body can and will naturally slim back down to that pre-set weight. If you go below your pre-set weight then the body will fight to return to the primal blueprint pre-set weight. But in fact the people who are unnaturally underweight will have an even harder battle to stay underweight than an overweight person will have to lose weight. Being underweight is unnatural and abnormal, returning to your natural ideal weight is a natural, normal state and in fact more easily achieved. The blueprint pattern for the perfect human body wasn't drawn and designed by the glamour mags for us all to aspire to and achieve.

'Repetition, repetition, repetition equals weight-loss success.'

Question: do you drink water? The answer is usually yes, but not enough. You may actually be drinking the correct quantity but it maybe the drinking style that's incorrect. I can see the puzzled look. People will often say that water makes them wee a lot, forever on the toilet; that is because they are drinking it in an incorrect fashion, in large amounts at random intervals, spasmodic. If you put a bowl of water down for a dog, what does it do? Does it A. drink a little and often, or B. drink the whole lot in one go? It drinks a little and often. People think that if they drink a pint of water in the morning and a pint of water in the afternoon, gulping it down as quickly as they can, then they have had their daily requirement of fluids. When you drink water quickly all that happens is the water is passed onto the bladder and the next place you visit is the toilet, with the water at best removing a few toxins. If you sip water throughout the day then it is absorbed by the body and used by the body. This is the correct way to drink, little and often. A leading consultant was attending my practice and when I asked him if he drank water his reply was yes, but not the recommended daily amount which is two litres. But think about this, if you drank two litres in the morning would this be your daily requirement? No, because most would be passed straight onto the bladder, benefiting the body little. Drinking has to be instinctive and variable depending on individual daily requirements. If it's a hot summer's day, you will require more water than on a freezing cold day in January. If you work out you will require more water than if you are relaxing with a good book. Drinking should be instinctive, variable and water should always be available. The consultant's reply was, "Yes you're right, people concentrate far too much on the quantity but not the quality of their drinking habits. So it's little and often you could say, but variable depending on the specific circumstances at the precise moment in time." A good system to make you aware of your thirst is to divide your day into six equal parts, I call this *'THE WATER SCALE OF HYDRATION:'* 1. morning, 2. mid-morning, 3. dinnertime, 4. mid-afternoon, 5. teatime, 6. after-tea. At these times become consciously aware of whether or not you have had a drink and spend a few minutes sipping water. This will then transpire to become a habit and will reignite instinctive drinking. Don't try to drown yourself with gallons, just sip. Water is the drink designed for the human body. The only reason why some people say that they don't like water is because the first drink given to a baby is usually some sugar-loaded juice drink, so from then on they drink for the taste of the sweetness of the sugar, making water then taste empty and boring in comparison. I know that not drinking water as water is meant to be drunk creates 50% of the world's obesity problem, maybe more. Water should be sipped regularly throughout the day, so that you don't confuse thirst pangs for hunger pangs. You will not suffer water retention. Water retention only happens when your body stores water because it can not rely on you to provide a constant supply. Your body cannot afford to be without water (the human body consists of 70% water, which needs maintaining), so if you are not providing a supply of pure fresh clear water, it has no other alternative but to store the water infrequently given. This also forces the body to use and recycle dirty water drawn from the bladder and the bowel. Water is a necessity for the human body. It needs a constant supply to lubricate the joints, maintain organ function and keep the body free from dehydration, as well as the thousands of other jobs water is required for in the general maintenance of a healthy human body. If your car's oil warning light flashes on do you take the bulb out or put oil into the engine? As most people will answer, you put oil into the engine obviously. If this is your answer but you are still not drinking enough water that means you are choosing to look after your car which can be easily replaced, but not your body which is irreplaceable – now there's a thought! If you don't supply the body with the water it needs, it will try to obtain it from food. This creates false hunger and eating food to satisfy thirst. Here lies a massive problem because if the food you are eating is dry as most processed food is then the amounts consumed could be colossal in the effort to obtain water from an impossible source. This is another reason why drinking water is imperative. If you had a life-threatening illness and by drinking water you would save your life, would you drink the water? I know your answer would be yes, of course. Well let me put this to you: water can stop you from contracting life-threatening illnesses and disabilities. Within three weeks of drinking water regularly you will notice a difference in your energy levels and general well-being. Water is the elixir of life and the only true drink. Every other feeds the body unnecessarily. Tea and coffee are diuretics so they actually make you wee more, but clinical reports show that tea and coffee do contain some beneficial properties. Two cups of coffee per day can give you a 35% less chance of becoming diabetic as the clinical trials, conducted at Harvard, have shown, as long as you still incorporate plain water into your daily routine. A glass of water more quickly drunk is beneficial for washing away toxins, but you still need to sip water throughout the day to avoid dehydration. Become accustomed to having a sip of water before a hot drink of tea or coffee! Alcohol, as well as other processed drinks, should be seen as a food rather than a drink. One 250ml glass of average strength red wine contains 214 calories. Two and a half glasses of wine can easily amount to one extra meal per day. Alcohol has no benefit to the human body and if you didn't force it into your body it would much prefer to be without. It learns to tolerate it, but that does not mean it is good for you, it just means you are giving your body no other alternative but to deal with it. Drink alcohol while you are enjoying the taste then stop, because if you are drinking to become drunk then you are drinking for reasons other than enjoying the drink itself and help is needed! Anyone who drinks by the clock at regular times each day, even if it only one small glass is, in my mind, an alcoholic. The alcohol is controlling the person not the person choosing the alcohol. If you must, then sip, taste, enjoy, but remember alcohol is not water or calorie free! Water is the only true drink! Don't see water as a tasteless boring drink, see it as nature's health-giving elixir: refreshing, energising and revitalising. Make the water bottle a modern-day fashion icon, take it with you everywhere you go, cool!

Before we go on to food, there are just a couple of notes worth a mention. First, food cravings are the intense desire to consume a specific food, and are stronger than normal hunger. This is to supply the body with what the body needs from that particular craved food type (notice the intense instinctive food cravings of pregnant women). As soon as the body has received the amount needed, the craving has served its purpose and dissipates. For example, a craving for strawberries signals a need for folate (folic acid, B9). These cravings should be short lived. Remember: cravings tell you what to eat, hunger tells you when to eat.

'The metabolism is essentially the amalgamation of

the sum of chemicals that react together within the human body.'

Second, people who are overweight will always state that they have a slow metabolism, while people classed as naturally thin will be said to have a fast metabolism. I believe that the human metabolism was set at the dawn of creation and works similarly to an automatic transmission: it slows down and speeds up depending on the conditions in which we live, depending how hard or how soft the human accelerator is pressed – it is variable. If we live in a world of 'fantasy famine' caused by restrictive dieting, then the metabolism will conserve fuel for human survival. If food is seen as always available, then fuel need not be conserved. However, by overeating, once again food is stored for the perceived 'fantasy famine' ahead. The secret to achieving and maintaining your natural ideal weight is to keep the body out of famine mode and this is achieved by eating food on bodily demand, hunger. The metabolism works like the accelerator on your car: Sleep/slow, exercise/fast. It controls the rate in which fuel is burned. If you are an overweight yo-yo dieter, you don't have a slow metabolic rate. You are just constantly living in famine mode triggered by nothing more than your own repetitive, restrictive fad diets themselves. You diet, enter famine mode, you fail; you diet, you fail. You never leave famine mode, because after a famine your body will conserve food/fuel for the next twelve weeks, which is longer than it takes the average yo-yo dieter to start the next restrictive vogue diet. I am sure that a large percentage of habitual restrictive dieters that enter famine mode on their very first diet will never again break free – biblical famines didn't last this long. We all have a metabolism that works relentlessly in conjunction with the person and their environment. If the environment is modified and fabricated while the metabolism remains true to its origins, then inevitably there will be an incompatible clash. Also something that is worth a mention is the hormone leptin. Hormones (which, when released, travel to another area in the body to make things happen) and endorphins (which function as neurotransmitters) are chemical messengers. Chemical imbalances that occur within the human body should themselves balance naturally when the body's natural equilibrium is restored and natural instinctive eating is reignited. As leptin is associated with weight loss, I feel it is worth knowing what it is and what it does. Leptin is king of the hormones; it is the commander-in-chief of virtually everything that takes place in the body. Leptin is made in the stored fat and acts as a gauge to keep the unconscious mind informed as to how much fuel is stored and available for use. This system works at its best when the body is at its natural ideal or optimum weight. When we become overweight, what appears to happen is that this direct line of communication becomes distorted. When we reduce our stored fat levels and become nearer to the body's natural ideal weight, the signals become more acutely clear. Leptin was discovered in 1994, so research into this hormone is still very much in its infancy, but it may be one of the more organic physical reasons why overweight people struggle to lose weight initially. But have heart, once stored fat starts to reduce communication will resume. Because leptin is produced within the stored fat, it increases when stored fat increases. It is as if a leptin traffic jam occurs (leptin resistance) in communication central. As fat reduces, the confusion clears and the system starts working as it should, with the signals then becoming definably clear. Obesity once again has been shown to cause unnatural, abnormal occurrences with in the human body. Removing the obstacle allows natural equilibrium to automatically restore. Other causes of obesity will, I am sure, be discovered in the future, but in a nutshell obesity is the cause of unnatural, abnormal balance within the human body. Once we become aware of this and rebalance by only supplying food/fuel when the body demands it, then the imbalances will no longer be there. It's hard living a natural life in a very unnatural world, but the mind-body connection, or in other words communication central, is still as functional today in each and everyone of us as it was yesterday and as it will be tomorrow.

'Food regulation/compensation is when we adjust what we eat to the physical activity we endure.'

There are only two types of food, primal-fresh (beneficial and good) and manufactured-processed (detrimental and not so good). How simple is that then? Fresh is best, as it contains fibre, vitamins, minerals, natural sugars, water and trace elements, all vital to the trouble-free running of a healthy human body. They contain all that is required for the human machine to faultlessly function with flawless perfection. Processed foods contain refined/processed sugar and eaten as the mainstay of a diet will induce obesity. Fresh foods are primal foods and the only foods your body was originally designed to eat, as water was to drink. Processed foods are foods not in their original natural state, as most if not all contain hidden sugars. These processed foods are all designed predominately for profit, and some manufacturers even mislead us into thinking they are genuinely healthy foods even though they are only masquerading as their primal superiors. One example of a processed food masquerading as a primal food is fruit juice drinks. Fruit is a primal food that is meant to be eaten and chewed and most definably not drunk as it is in its mutated processed form. Fruit juice creates a concentrated sugar overload, as healthy sugars like fructose become unhealthy in their processed form causing a metabolic catastrophe. So eat your fruit as it was always meant to be! A mother will be led into believing that beans on toast are a healthy choice for their children, as what mother would give a child knowingly unhealthy foods. She has been told and now believes that beans are healthy and so they are in their natural unmodified state, such as broad beans, runner beans, kidney beans and haricot beans. However baked beans are processed haricot beans. All the natural life force and goodness is lost in the processing, and then worse still they are loaded with taste-addictive, refined/processed sugar. Sugar should be considered as addictive as class 'A' drugs. These sugars are classed as hidden sugars, so when a mother gives her child beans on toast, she is unaware that she is exposing her child to the high dosage of sugar in a tin of baked beans. So then the child will ask, when given a choice of what to have for tea, for beans on toast, please. Mum thinks beans, healthy; but the child is only asking for them because of their growing addiction to the sweet taste of the sugars. Everything going according to the food marketers plan, as this is exactly what is meant to happen – devious or what! We become conditioned and manipulated by the big food companies. Just think about this example of a tea consisting of beans on toast:

A tin of baked beans contains processed beans in a thick sugar sauce = SUGAR.

Bread = carbohydrate = starch = SUGAR.

A glass of fizzy pop = SUGAR.

After tea, a sweet, pudding, cakes, biscuits = SUGAR.

So you may just as well give your child a 2 lb bag of sugar and a lollipop and say, get stuck in.

'Hidden sugar added to food is unethical!'

Sugar can be disguised with over fifty different names, so making healthy choices is not as straightforward as at first it seems. We are often subject to deception and misdirection in our purchases. I am not saying don't ever eat processed food. I, like you, enjoy beans on toast, but not at every meal. The key is everything in moderation. The foods that are good for us, that is, the ones that the human body was designed to consume to create optimum performance, are foods that are in their natural unprocessed state. In fact, if you want to know what to eat consult a caveman! Imagine what he would eat because that will be the correct, compatible and complementary food to sustain a healthy human body. But the problem posed is this: the world has evolved, but the human body has not. It still needs the designer's fuel of choice as written in the original manual. Food today is designed for profit and not always with the priority of human health in mind. You will tolerate it, but that is not to say it is good for you. With today's modern families all too often under extreme pressure from work commitments in order to maintain an acceptable standard of living, choosing easy to prepare processed foods over unprocessed primal foods after an hard day at the office is commonplace. This could be seen as body-negligence only to purchase the latest media technology or must have fad-gadget. So where do your priories lie? Put as much effort into the choice of your food as you would into the purchase of a new car, because the car can be easily replaced, you can't! A lot of the processed foods we eat are being sold legally mislead customers for profit; baked beans are a prime example. Because we have been told that beans are good for us, we now associate and accept any beans as good. We have to open our eyes, ask questions, and understand what is really good for our bodies and what is just twisted misleading information for the big food companies profits! The human body has a natural food tolerance. That does not mean that certain specific foods are good for us, it just means that we can tolerate them. We are told for example that meat is good for us and that it makes us strong, but I'm not sure. Don't think for one minute I am preaching vegetarianism, I'm not! I think meat was eaten in the caveman era for survival, while fresh fruits and vegetables became available again throughout the summer months. That does not mean it was good for him, it just means he tolerated it to preserve human life in times of food scarcity. Also meat would not be caught every day. The same applies to milk. Name another animal that drinks milk after being weaned from its mother, you can't. Milk is designed for babies; still to this day no superior manufactured substitute for same species milk has been formulated to supply offspring necessities, and it never will. The strongest and biggest land mammal in the world is the elephant, a vegetarian, non-meat-eating animal; how strong do you want to be? Also it has the biggest teeth, the tusks, of any living land mammal and never drinks a drop of milk for calcium after being weaned from its mother. So many questions that need to be asked never are. Now is the time to ask. It's your health that's at risk. The next generation has to be a generation of inquisitive Bamber Gascoigne's (now that shows my age) digging out all the answers to unearth the buried truths.

'30% of all your daily water intake should come from the food you eat.'

Just one final note: the first thing dieters do when they start a diet is cut out sugar altogether, instantly. Now, remember sugar is more addictive than class 'A' drugs, so inevitably if you cut sugar out altogether your body will crave it, because it's become used to receiving it and to some degree it has learnt to rely on it in an expectant fashion. A small amount of sugar harms no one, that single piece of cake was never responsible for you being overweight. Remember to eat when your hungry and stop when your satisfied. Don't eat for environmental cues and reasons other than hunger. Most importantly, enjoy your food and eat everything in moderation. If someone told me that I should never have another piece of cake I know I would, so would you. Don't set yourself targets that are impossible to meet, as that's exactly what you have done in the past. Retraining the mind to listen to the hunger and satiety signals compares best to learning to ride a bike. You start off with stabilisers and when confidence is built up, they are removed and you fall off. If you don't jump right back on you will never learn to ride the bike. See mistakes as part of learning to attain the desired success! We have to challenge our core belief system and explore whether or not we have consciously chosen them. Most of our beliefs have been instilled in us by the people we love, verbally or non-verbally. The same people who would be devastated to know the pain caused by these fallacious beliefs. Most children are brought up with dieting playing a predominant part in their parent's lives, especially their mum's, then reflected in theirs. They come to believe that the only way to lose weight is by food restriction and food deprivation. Depriving the body of food when food is needed and signalled by hunger damages the body through malnutrition, producing serious conditions. That's why it is just as important to eat when hungry as it is to stop when satisfied and it is imperative to supply the correct nutrients to satisfy the bodies fundamental requirements, found mainly only in primal, unprocessed foods. Obesity is a chronic condition, with the world's population suffering weight loss neurosis fuelled by the pressure of unrealistic media expectations and the unreliable diet industry itself. Even the gyms and their trainers promote exercise for weight loss. This is no different than the diet clubs promoting their restrictive diets, as it does, as it always will, end in failure. Exercise is cardiovascular, muscular and body sculpting; beneficial with the correct advice. Weight loss begins with what goes into the mouth. If we exercise and restrict calorie intake, weight loss will fail. This is bad for clients but good for gyms with all those unused memberships adding to profits. Most diet and weight loss groups rely heavily on fear and shame to achieve any degree of *weight-loss success.* You pay your £5 per week, what for? Only to be weighed. This creates fear of not losing weight and shame of gaining weight, so people will resort to the most severe levels of food deprivation and restriction to lose weight before the weigh-in. This suggests to the attendee *weight-loss success,* even though mostly, you know, it will only be short lived. 'Slimming foods' contain no magic ingredients different to what you would normally cook yourself, the difference is in the portion sizes. You pay however many times more for something that you could easily cook yourself and just eat less of, saving the rest for tomorrow; mind tricks and psychological misdirection comes to mind. *Warning:* don't aggressively exercise until your weight is reduced. Why? Think about it. You weigh nineteen stones and you rigorously exercise, you may in fact be causing irreversible and permanent damage to all of your joints due to the fact that they were never originally designed to carry such an unnatural, abnormal amount of weight. A brisk walk is all you need; walking one step quicker than would normally feel comfortable. Whatever is said, fat does not and will not transfer into muscle. It's a myth. Fat reduces and muscle gains and fat will continue to reduce without exercise when natural instinctive eating is reignited. And jogging, why? *J.S.J*, Jogging Shatters Joints. It also makes you look a *N.O.B*, exactly! Either run, walk or mix the two, but never jog, it's just so wrong! It's my opinion that Keys proved in the 1950s that restrictive diets don't work. This has been confirmed only recently by a retired boss of one of the more well-known and dominant multi-billion pound diet clubs, stating on national TV that their business relies mainly on customer failure for their own success. I'll tell you now that there is no magic pill, just a responsibility that lies totally with you! Don't let the Dick Turpin's of the diet industry steal all of your hard-earned cash. It should be you saying, "Stand and deliver," but they can't and probably never will!

'With every gram of fat you store, you store four grams of water. Don't become a walking reservoir.'

Talk Yourself Slim With The Self Chatter Diet enables you to recognise and realise your own detrimental beliefs, behaviours and associations by creating a clear self-insight and awareness, so that you can then make all the changes necessary to achieve your own *weight-loss success.* Here ends the logical approach. Read it through a few more times until it is fully understood. Each time you read it you will form a deeper understanding within the unconscious mind. Then move on to the next chapter where I discuss the systematic method and how it is to be effectively applied. But always remember to question and challenge and never be afraid of asking the question, why?

'History will be kind to me for I intend to write it.'

Winston Churchill

Remember, it doesn't have to be this way forever!

CHAPTER THREE

TALK YOURSELF SLIM WITH THE SELF-CHATTER DIET: A SYSTEMATIC METHOD TO ACHIEVE WEIGHT-LOSS SUCCESS

As a man thinketh in his heart, so is he.

The main difference between the two minds, the conscious mind and the unconscious mind, is that we know what the conscious mind is thinking, therefore the conscious mind is us ('The I mind') and the fundamental reason why we have become the most supreme species to have ever walked on the face of the earth due to an unmatchable ability to respond to an original idea or unusual situation in an analytical intellectual way. Whereas, the unconscious mind is, in its thinking, only the sum total of our primal genetic instincts, but most importantly, our past experiences intellectually analysed or not by the conscious mind – ('The Animalistic Mind').

As a child, and before the critical faculty of the conscious mind is reliably formed, information is taken literately and all to often is misinterpreted with the unconcious mind arriving at its own erroneous internal conclusion. This provides a fertile ground for fallacious limiting beliefs to grow, such as the breakfast, dinner and tea general pattern of behaviour. These fallacious limiting beliefs stop the body from achieving and maintaining its primal blueprint pre-set weight. Any action repeated over and over again soon becomes a learnt behaviour or a habitual auto-behaviour, or, simply put, a habit. If the foundations of the habit are based on the fallacious limiting belief that breakfast, dinner and tea should never be missed at whatever cost, then the habit formed becomes as good as fact as far as the unconscious mind is concerned, even though it is detrimental to the human body. The unconscious mind will never again intellectually question or challenge the belief, it will only respond rigorously and relentlessly to the triggered associations of 8am, 1pm and 5.30pm, resulting in food dictation. Breakfast, dinner and tea is the rogue programme that in the main leads to all that consists in the formation of human obesity. We have to change our core belief system and recognise and realise (self-insight) the habits that accompany the associations that produce the detrimental actions that create obesity. We have to change our cognition, that is, the way in which we process our thoughts into knowledge and where the inner voice of self-chatter plays a fundamental part of changing these beliefs, behaviours and associations. We have to identify, then intellectually question and challenge these beliefs by using the inner voice of self-chatter. We can then, by deliberate conscious intent, change the core (limiting) belief system and form new beneficially constructive and proactive beliefs, behaviours and associations built on undistorted fact. The new formed habits (responding actions) will then become normalised, resulting in long-term *weight-loss success: following 'The Master Programme'.*

'Obesity is a chronic behavioural condition.'

No-one can lose weight for you. I, the author, have no magical powers and can give you no magic pill. The reality is that its all down to you: the desire to change is of paramount importance to *weight-loss success.* The desire to change is the greatest of all human motivators to bring change about. We have to question and challenge our core (limiting) belief system and habitual auto-behaviours along with all the associations connected by forming an internal locus of control. That is, you are responsible for your own actions, behaviours, outcomes and successes. The method showing to be most successful in producing cognitive change is by the use of the inner voice of self-chatter. By internally vocalising we can recognise and realise our beliefs, behaviours and associations (self-insight), questioning and challenging them. By keeping our eating behaviours (actions) consciously mindful we can successfully bring about the necessary changes, producing a successful outcome. It's how the inner voice of self-chatter is incorporated within the systematic method of *Talk Yourself Slim With The Self-Chatter Diet* that is proving, in my opinion, to be the most effective method in facilitating these changes: the optimised systematic method to *weight-loss success.*

'Let hunger motivate not the environment dictate.'

THE METHOD TO APPLY

This is the fun part of the systematic method, as now the time has come to let your imagination run riot. Imagination is the language of the unconscious mind, so the more creativity you add to the images created the more profound the effect will be. You must remember in the process to use all of your five senses. So unleash your mind and let your imagination come out to play!

Relax in your favourite chair or lie on your bed. First, I want you to imagine your stomach as something identifiable. The image you generate can be anything from the weird and wacky and the totally outrageous to Mr Sensible, the local librarian. It can take the form of your favourite film star or TV personality, a pet you love or an animal of your choice, a wise one from Mahatma Gandhi to Albus Dumbledore, from Buddha to Elvis, maybe someone you love and admire, to a cartoon character remembered from childhood (Scooby Doo and He-Man were favourites of mine). It's not who or what the identifiable image looks like but the image itself that's imperative – *an image*. Now the image needs a name. If the image you have created already has a name, then use that one; if not, give it one. You could even give your image a name badge or see the name clearly tattooed on the person's forehead. Now let the name resonate deep within your mind. Repeat the name over and over, focusing on your chosen image until you become comfortability familiar with it, as now this created image is your new best friend!

Now the image of your stomach has been created and named. From now on before you eat even one piece of food, always first ask this image by its name, using your inner voice of self-chatter, "Am I hungry?" Always trust the instant and intuitive answer it gives and respond accordingly with the appropriate action. When eating, always eat consciously and mindfully, enjoying every mouthful: feel the textures, enjoy the flavours. Allow your choice of food to be nourishing, nutritious and healthy, with primal foods making up the staple part of your daily diet; that is, foods in their natural state, unmodified by processing. Remember as well to drink adequate amounts of water. It is the only drink that is not a food, every other is! Eat until your new best friend, your chosen image, is satisfied, and imagine them saying, "That's enough, thank you very much, I'm satisfied, *stop now*!" With time and practice the signals will become loud and clear, so fake it until you make it by trusting your own intuition and your body's inner-wisdom.

By using the inner voice of self-chatter you become consciously aware of whether or not you are eating because of genuine hunger or because of something else. Once questioned and challenged, if your 'hunger' is because of something else (phantom hunger), then do something else, preferably something enjoyable to you; if it is genuine hunger, eat. These habitual auto-behaviours along with corresponding triggered associations and the detrimental fallacious core belief system upon which they were once formed is soon rendered inactive. By using the inner voice of self-chatter we can, by deliberate conscious intent, replace these behaviours and allow new beneficially constructive and proactive ones to become normalised by the unconscious mind as it forms new habitual auto-behaviours and corresponding triggered associations that are built on a new and reliable belief; with hunger becoming the trigger (the association) for the response to eat (the behaviour). In this way we acknowledge and become aware of the detrimental behaviours that are causing obesity, and that it is only by recognising, realising, questioning and challenging these behaviours that we are able to change and supersede them. By using the inner voice of self-chatter, or self-talk, we keep consciously mindful of these behaviours, thus enabling change. This process lets us **A**cknowledge, **R**eprogramme and **S**ucceed – *weight-loss success!*

THE 'SECRET' OF TALK YOURSELF SLIM WITH THE SELF-CHATTER DIET.

To reignite natural instinctive eating, you have to first ACKNOWLEDGE – ask your inner voice, am I hungry or is it something else? Secondly, REPROGRAMME – responding accordingly to the inner voice's answer. Thirdly, SUCCEED – the conscious action will change the unconscious programme.

We are the sum of our thoughts and our thoughts are very powerful in the effects they cause. Changing the way in which we talk to ourselves, our thoughts and way of thinking, we can change limiting beliefs, learnt behaviours, habitual auto-behaviours and corresponding triggered associations. At (approx.) twelve years old, intelligence is formed fully enough to analyse incoming information in a more reliable manner and store information (knowledge) according to its true meaning. When we create a mental image or picture, it burns into the hard-drive of the unconscious mind, because *imagination is the language of the unconscious mind* – read this statement again. This becomes a belief. This belief then causes a response to future situations. If the response is repeated over and over again it will become a habit, creating and attaching corresponding triggered associations, as a habit is the repetition of an action. Essentially, we must change the belief system that dictates, 'I must eat breakfast every morning before I leave the house', or even, 'If I leave the house without breakfast, I will die', to 'I eat breakfast if I'm hungry and I don't eat breakfast if I'm not'. This is a new beneficially constructive and proactive belief. Changing our behaviours is no different than reprogramming a computer to perform a different task. If you don't input the information then the computer will continue to follow the old programme. We are no different. We are following out-of-date, unreliable data that was programmed before we had acquired enough knowledge to vet all incoming information in accordance to its true intention (not always the literal) for future reference and response.

> 'EMOTIONAL EATING IS NOTHING
> MORE THAN TRIGGERED
> ASSOCIATIONS MADE PASSIVE
> THROUGH REALISATION'

So by using the inner voice of self-chatter as part of the *Talk Yourself Slim With The Self-Chatter Diet,* we keep focused and mindful of our eating behaviours. We can then recognise and realise (self-insight) detrimental habits and make cognitive changes that replace those behaviours that stop us from achieving *weight-loss success.* After a period of time, the inner voice of self-chatter will calm and the behaviours will become normalised. Natural instinctive eating will become as normal as breathing. A new pattern of behaviour will have been created, a new belief forming positive, beneficially constructive and proactive learnt behaviours, habitual auto-behaviours and associations. Hunger and satiety signals will now replace taking meals by the clock or food dictation. The repetition of an action forms a habit, so by repeatedly listening to bodily signals (the cybernetic loop – the mind-body connection) instead of environmental cues (breakfast, dinner and tea) we reignite natural instinctive eating and allows the body's intelligence to regulate and compensate its food intake and fat storage. However, this behaviour cannot be changed until it is recognised, realised, questioned and challenged, until we are made consciously aware and strive to replace it by deliberate intent. Until obesity is addressed as being a behavioural issue, and treated as such, no solution will ever be found. This is because food is not the prime cause of obesity but the behavioural manner in which food is eaten!

THE FIVE BASIC PRINCIPALS OF TALK YOURSELF SLIM WITH THE SELF-CHATTER DIET THE SYSTEMATIC

METHOD TO ACHIEVING WEIGHT-LOSS SUCCESS

1. To recognise, realise question and challenge your core (limiting) beliefs, learnt behaviours or habitual auto-behaviours and all their corresponding triggered associations that will lead you into obesity, taking full responsibility for your actions, behaviours, outcomes and successes and therefore forming an internal locus of control – Julian Rotter – Locus of Control of Reinforcement – 1950s.

2. Consciously, with intent and deliberately by choice, change your core (limiting) beliefs, learnt behaviours or habitual auto-behaviours along with all their corresponding triggered associations and as a consequence, reignite natural instinctive eating, resulting in *weight-loss success*. Return the unconscious mind, the programme, to a pattern of responding and reacting to the body's natural hunger and satiety signals. This is part of the body's intelligence or the cybernetic loop, the mind-body connection, which should not be dictated to by unnaturally manufactured and fabricated environmental cues or predicted eating and food-dictation.

3. The inner voice of self-chatter helps you maintain a constant conscious awareness of your own individual eating habits. By becoming consciously aware of your own core (limiting) beliefs, learnt behaviours or habitual auto-behaviours and their corresponding triggered associations, you can replace one behaviour with another, using conscious intent. The optimum result is the reignition of natural instinctive eating. By repeating an action, the new behaviour soon becomes a normalised response to genuine hunger and satiety signals, variable by nature, not dictated by time, otherwise known as weight-loss success.

4. Primal foods should form the mainstay of all human diet. The key is to eat foods that would have existed during the Palaeolithic era. During this period, and before the introduction of agriculture, humans had no other choice but to hunt and gather their food. All foods consumed came directly from nature. With the introduction of agricultural and later industrial ages, the human diet changed to include grains, sugars and processed foods. It's believed that this change in diet is responsible for diseases like heart disease, high blood pressure and cancer, as the human body is simply not genetically engineered to eat modified foods. Build your diet around primal foods, that is, foods in their

natural unprocessed state, foods compatible to the human design, just as nature intended.

5. Water is the elixir of life. Water is the only true drink, as everything else feeds the body and doesn't serve the purpose intended. The human body depends on a constant supply of water of which it is now generally denied. Water keeps the body in a healthy state and must be reinstated as the drink of life, to eradicate early human demise. Early wear and tear is connected with insufficient water acting as a lubricant to joints and feeding organs to avoid dysfunction and failure. Water is essential in the general running of the human machine.

'TALK YOURSELF SLIM WITH THE SELF-CHATTER DIET, CONQUERING MAN'S NEMESIS.'

CHAPTER FOUR

M.I.R – WHAT IS MIND IMAGERY REPROGRAMMING?

'The thoughts in your mind become the things in your hand.'

M.I.R: *Mind Imagery Reprogramming is a technique to facilitate change.* Evolved, developed and adapted at The Feelbetterfast Clinic by the author of these works, Mr. John Richardson, to facilitate change within the programme of the unconscious mind responsible for our core beliefs, learnt behaviours or habitual auto-behaviours along with all corresponding triggered associations, based on the understanding that imagination is the language of the unconscious mind. This is a technique that produces rapid and amazing results; used with an operator or self.

Your thoughts are very powerful, more powerful than you can ever imagine. Thoughts will produce physical reactions within the human body, so what and how you think is very important to your health and well-being. Imagination is the language of the unconscious mind, what you imagine does tend to happen or become your reality. Whenever imagination and logic are in conflict, imagination usually wins the day (Coue's Law of Reversed Effort).

Imagine you find a lump on your body, instantly you think the worst. You make an appointment with your local GP, but what if the receptionist says that he cannot see you for three days? Those three days are the longest three days of your life. By the time you arrive for your appointment you have imagined all the uncomfortable treatments that you have to endure, the hospital where you will be given your treatments at and probably even your own funeral. These negative thoughts will cause your body to react as though the illness is real, whether it is or not. This is because the unconscious mind cannot tell the difference between something that is imagined and something that is real and will respond equally the same to both situations. When the GP tells you that it's nothing more than a cyst, you nearly kiss him with relief. You walk into the surgery as though any time you're about to take your last breath and leave doing cartwheels, all with a change of your thoughts – powerful!

Preconceived ideas will continuously keep the human body in a state of apprehension, especially if you are of a fearful nature. This being the chief instigator in the activation of the fight or flight response causing a person to act with irrational and neurotic behaviours, for what at first appears to have no apparent reason.

Imagination is used throughout the day, when you remember a past experience, think of someone you know or when you daydream. We have all been for a job interview and imagined the outcome before the interview has even taken place, or been late for work and imagined how the boss was going to react. These are all forms of you using your imagination.

Entering the 'alpha state' through relaxation and visualisation allows imagined positive, deliberate by intent, suggestions to enter the unconscious mind without conscious analytical intervention, so that the unconscious mind (your programme) and conscious mind (intelligence) can communicate in a positive way without other external forces intruding, concentrating only on the present tense imagined suggestions. We can use imagination while in the 'alpha state' or 'alpha-relaxation' to change old tapes; limiting beliefs, learnt behaviours or habitual auto-behaviours and triggered associations. Imagination burns a mental picture into the unconscious mind and once that picture is there your unconscious mind gets to work at making that picture your reality. Once an idea has been accepted by the unconscious mind it will remain there until it is replaced by another idea. Your unconscious mind cannot hold on to two concepts of the same idea, so once a new idea has been accepted, the old idea will modify or disappear. It will be replaced by the new imagined and deliberately intended appropriate one. The longer the idea remains the more opposition there is to replacing it with another new idea. This is *Mind Imagery Reprogramming* or *M.I.R,* the use of imagination with positive deliberate intent.

Using *Mind Imagery Reprogramming* or *M.I.R.* the imagination is deliberate, creating mental images consciously for change. The difference between our dreams and our imagination is that dreams are unconscious whereas the imagination can be used consciously to evoke and promote change. Using *Mind Imagery Reprogramming* the images are consciously created and burnt into the unconscious mind. The more intense, specific and descriptive the created images are the more impact they will have on the unconscious mind effecting the end result. Dreams have no conscious control, whereas imagination has.

Imagination is not just pictured images as some believe, it involves all the five senses. Some people will be more receptive to one of the five scenes and this will become the more prominent part of their imagination. One thing to remember is this: everyone can imagine, we all use it in our everyday life as part of the recall of memories. For example, what colour is your front door? Now your thinking (imagination recall), then you say, blue or whatever the colour of your door is. Next I ask you, which side of the door is the handle on? I bet you will instantly put your hand out and imagine opening the door (imagination recall) and say, this side. This is a perfect example of imagination recall, when we use imagination to recall information from the unconscious mind. Then there is creative imagination. Creative imagination is when we see something before it has been created. These are the people that usually perform well in a stage hypnosis show, sometimes classed as the 'Walter Mittys' of the world, the dreamers, the fantasisers. Not everyone has a dominant originative creative imagination, but everyone has imagination recall, though most lay somewhere in between. Once an idea becomes accepted by the unconscious mind, that idea becomes fact. The unconscious mind is very clever, but not intelligent, so it does not analyse. If everything appears as it should be, the programme will run, no questions asked. Always remember the golden rule: imagination is the language of the unconscious mind.

When using *Mind Imagery Reprogramming* the eyes remain closed throughout as the body enters 'alpha-relaxation'. The eyes are closed to shut out the outside world and to open up the inside world, removing external distractions. By relaxing and entering the 'alpha state' or 'alpha-relaxation' the mind becomes more receptive to the imagination. Relaxation is the single most important aspect of *Mind Imagery Reprogramming – M.I.R,* because effective use of the imagination takes place when the mind is in the 'alpha state'. This state occurs naturally when the body becomes very relaxed, induced with the use of visualisation induction techniques and deepeners. Relaxation is a great healer in its own right. It returns a person to a natural balance in which the body can heal itself and the mind is at peace. The relaxation response is at the opposite pole to the fight or flight response and counteracts its effect.

Using imagination is not only visual as stated earlier. The visual component is usually the strongest, but all the senses must and should be used to the best of your ability. Vision is most people's strongest sense, but another sense will be more dominant in some. When an emotion is added to imagination, the image is strengthened ten-fold.

When using *Mind Imagery Reprogramming,* whether on yourself or another, it is always important to focus on what you want to happen and not what you don't. On things you want, and not the things you have but don't want. If you remain focused on what you have, then the unconscious mind will maintain that as your ongoing reality. You should always be thinking about and imagining what you really want so that the unconscious mind will start to work right away on making that your new reality. See yourself as you want to be, right now! Ignore your present reality for a while and imagine the life desired, instead of what you have that is undesired. Tap into the emotions of how that new life would feel if you had it right now. Be specific when using imagination. Imagine through your own eyes, you being the star of the show, the main character. Using daily affirmations will keep the mind focused on the goal. It's good to use affirmations first thing in the morning and last thing at night, just after and just before sleep. In the morning, the mind is fresh and receptive, it is not busy dealing with the daily problems of everyday life. Using affirmations just before sleep will leave the mind all night to work on the ideas imagined – affirmations can never be overused and their potential is endless!

> *'The life you are experiencing today is the result of your previous thoughts, feelings and actions. The life you will experience tomorrow will be the result of your thoughts, feelings and actions today. Remember, as you think today, so tomorrow will be.'*

My grandfather J. Arthur Laundon always told me as a small boy to go to sleep on a good thought. He would say, "Let the last thought you have before you go to sleep be a positive one, like, when I wake up in the morning I will feel fantastic." Repeat this or another over and over before you drift off into a peaceful slumber, it works miracles.

Mind Imagery Reprogramming – M.I.R, is the use of imagination while in the 'alpha state' or 'alpha-relaxation' to communicate with the unconscious mind without other conscious intervention, only focused intent, to bring about necessary changes by removing the obstacles that stop us from achieving and reaching our goals. Imagination will only win over logic 100% of the time.

Mind Imagery Reprogramming – M.I.R, is a fast and effective way to reset the human computer, recalibrate the mind's programme and form stronger communications within the mind-body connection, reigniting natural instinctive eating and achieving *weight-loss success.*

M.I.R.™- MIND IMAGERY REPROGRAMMING; IMPLANTING THE NEW REMOVING THE OLD

ACHIEVING THE 'ALPHA STATE' OR 'ALPHA-RELAXATION' FOR THE SUCCESSFUL UTILISATION OF MIND IMAGERY REPROGRAMMING – M.I.R – TO FACILITATE CHANGE BY CONTROLLED DELIBERATE INTENT

The induction of the 'alpha state' or 'alpha-relaxation' is a simple process which improves with practice. I have found that this progressive fractional relaxation technique is a simple yet effective way to achieve the desired objective. Start by making yourself comfortable, either sitting or laying comfortably, dim the light, maybe play some soft music, and be sure you will not be disturbed for the allotted time, then start with this simple repetitive fractional relaxation sequence:

Take three deep breaths and on each of the out breaths think, relax, then:

- Relax the scalp area from the top of your head down to the nape of your neck.
- Relax your forehead.
- Relax your eyes.
- Relax your cheekbones.
- Relax your jaw and mouth (allow your teeth and lips to become slightly parted).
- Relax your neck and shoulders.
- Relax your upper arms, your elbows, your forearms, and down to your hands and fingers.
- Relax your back and chest area.
- Relax your abdominal area.
- Relax your hip and pelvic area.
- Relax your thigh muscles.
- Relax your knees.
- Relax your calf muscles.
- Relax your feet and toes
- Count down from 10 to 0 – repeat the sequence two

or three times (or more if required) prior to all Mind Imagery Reprogramming M.I.R – visualisation. The scripts and techniques presented here can be chopped, changed and adapted to suit the individual's requirements and be creative, always focusing on what you want. You are the story…

Script technique 1: Imagine, really imagine, that you are now walking along a road, a long straight road that ends in a T-junction with one road leading off to the left and one road leading off to the right. The left road leads to a life of obesity, misery, ill health and a short life. It is a short road, and a very short journey – a Dead Man's Road! The right road leads to a life of you being at your natural ideal weight, good health and a long and happy life. It's a long road, and a very long journey – Longevity Lane! Feel the road under your feet as you walk briskly towards the junction. And now imagine that you are standing at the junction with a very important choice to make, but remember the choice is yours, it's for you to make. As you stand on the junction with this very important choice to make, the most important choice that in your life you will ever have to make, of which road will you take, remember always that the choice is yours. It is a choice that only you can decide upon. But before you make this choice, let's take a look at the consequences of both these two choices that you have before you and see how they can and will determine and effect the rest of your life, your future.

First, I want you to imagine life five, ten, fifteen, twenty years from now. You haven't lost the weight, you've put even more on. You're in a bedroom, in the bedroom there is a bed, a table and a chair, a window, a TV, by the bed there is an oxygen bottle and folded in the corner of the room a wheelchair – these are yours. You have all the ailments that accompany being overweight: diabetes, high risk of heart attacks and strokes, hypertension, cholesterol, breathing difficulties, mysterious aches and pains, and the list goes on and it's not pretty. You don't go out much because you are totally dependant on other people taking you, but other people make excuses so you get left home alone. This is not living, it's only existing. You're not enjoying your family, you're not enjoying your friends, but most importantly you are not enjoying your life. This is not a nice feeling. Now I want you to forget this scenario, because this is not going to be your choice, this is not going to be an option. Let's see how it's going to be, how it has to be, how it will be.

Imagine, five, ten, fifteen, twenty years from now and

you have lost the weight, you look fantastic, you feel fantastic. You're not trapped in a bedroom, you're out there enjoying life. All the ailments have disappeared, melted away, and you feel on top of the world. You don't rely on someone taking you out, you take other people out. No oxygen bottle needed here, no wheelchair required and you are doing all the things that you want to do. You are enjoying your family, you are enjoying your friends and most importantly you are now enjoying your life. You are fifty looking thirty acting sixteen, now this is the nice feeling.

I want you now to take your mind back once again to the junction where you are waiting to make this very important choice, and remember that the choice is yours. It always has been, it always will be; it's for you to make. The left road leads to a life of obesity, misery, ill health. It's a short road and a very short journey, you can actually see the end in sight. The right road leads to a life of being at your natural ideal weight, good health, and a long and happy life. It's a long road and a very long journey, the end is nowhere in sight. The road goes on for miles and miles. As always the choice is yours, only you can decide. See yourself now making that very important choice, the choice that will effect the rest of your life. Imagine making the right choice and walking down the right road, the road that is your choice. Imagine your family, your friends, your children (if applicable) waving, beckoning you down the right road. You walk, then run down that road. Imagine the feeling that this gives you. It is a feeling that you never want to let go of, a feeling that you now know you can very easily achieve, because you know that you can be anything you want to be. You've taken the right road, made the right choice and you are now enjoying the journey and this feels fantastic. You are now walking on the sunny side of the street to *weight-loss success!* You are a very important person to your family, to your friends, to your children. If something happened to you, something that you could have easily avoided, just imagine how they would feel. Visiting you lying in a hospital bed or worse still lying on a cold mortuary slab, and all because you didn't listen to your body. You actually thought you knew best. The doctors have proven that organs taken from overweight people show signs of being larger and stronger. That's because they are having to work twice as hard. Logic says that if they are having to work twice as hard, then they will and often do wear out twice as quick. This is not good, but this is also not you. You have achieved *weight-loss success!* Return to the here and now when the time feels right for you by counting from 1 to 5, then saying, "I'm now wide awake and feeling fine, let battle commence."

'VISUALISE A NEW SLIMMER YOU.'

Script technique 2: Imagine, and really imagine, your heart. Imagine it as a little animated cartoon character; imagine it with a sad face and dripping from head to toe in white, gooey, sticky fat. This little heart loves you: it knows it has to beat to keep you alive, and it knows that if it stops then you die. But what it doesn't understand is why you allow it to be smothered in white, gooey, sticky fat, making its job twice as hard and at times almost impossible. The same applies to all your organs, they are all drowning in a sea of white, gooey, sticky fat. Your heart works seven days a week, fifty-two weeks a year with no time off, and what thanks do you give it? None! You just force it to work even harder and harder. How much do you think it can take? It's slave labour; it's all work with no play. Everyone and everything has a breaking point. It's just a matter of time. If you were walking up a big steep hill on a hot summer's day wearing a big thick winter coat you would stop and take that coat off, making your life as easy as possible. Your heart can't do this on it's own. It relies totally on you, just like all your other organs. If you cleaned the windows on the outside of your house, you wouldn't leave the inside dirty. You have an outside and you have an inside. It's clear to see that you look after and maintain the outside very well, I just wonder what the inside looks like. If you didn't have your car serviced, if you didn't look after it, take care of it, then one day the engine would let you down. Your body is your vehicle, if you don't look after your body then one day your organs, your engine, will let you down. Your body is designed to live 100 years in a state of perfect health, we disable our bodies through negligence, ignorance, carelessness, a lack of responsibility and at times even laziness, then when something goes wrong we panic and wonder why. Should we really wonder? Obesity is the slowest form of suicide. It is a long drawn out process of illness and disease leading to eventual death. You have put obstacles in the way of your health, simply by removing these obstacles you can once again easily return and restore your body to perfect health. It's no good wishing tomorrow that you had made the changes today, because tomorrow will come. Simply remove the obstacle and achieve the goal of perfect health. Now imagine and really imagine your heart looking like Mr (or Miss) Universe or your favourite film star: fit and healthy, all the white, gooey, sticky fat gone and in its place rippling muscle as it deals with its daily chores with ease and comfort. Then imagine the whole inside of your body, with all your organs looking brand spanking new, no sign of visceral fat and every organ functioning efficiently, and effectively. You have achieved *weight-loss success!* Return to the here and now when the time feels right for you by counting from 1 to 5, then saying, "I'm now wide awake and feeling fine, let battle commence."

'IMAGINE YOU ARE NOW THE PERSON YOU WANT TO BE.'

Script technique 3: Imagine, and really imagine, that right in front of you is a dustbin. Inside the dustbin are cakes and buns, biscuits, crisps, sweets and chocolate, junk foods, processed foods, and the bin is topped up to the brim with alcohol. In your hands you have a big wooden spoon and you are now stirring all the ingredients together into a thick creamy, gooey mixture. Feel yourself turning it and stirring it mixing all the ingredients together with the big wooden spoon, knocking all the lumps out until it is a smooth and thick creamy, gooey mixture. In the mixture, as you stir, rotting fish guts, fish heads and maggots begin to appear. The rotting smell is rising up your nose and going down into the back of your throat, you retch, but you keep mixing, turning and stirring. In your pocket you have a teaspoon, you take the teaspoon out from your pocket as you are now going to sample this mixture. You dip the spoon into the mixture and put the mixture onto your tongue. The rotting smell drifts up your nose and down your throat, you retch again. Now, you have a choice, you can either swallow the mixture and it will seriously damage and destroy your body, or you can simply spit it out: you do have a choice, so what are you going to do? That's right, go on spit it out. Remember to make sure the maggot that slipped under your tongue has also come out! But you will never forget that smell or that taste. Now see food exactly for what it really is, fuel for your body, and your body deserves only the best, the very best. Eating is not a hobby, it is fuelling your body, you have achieved *weight-loss success!* (This is also a very effective 'specific food' aversion technique; using the 'specific food' in the mixture). Return to the here and now when the time feels right for you by counting from 1 to 5, then saying, "I'm now wide awake and feeling fine, let battle commence."

'IMAGINE ON A BOTTLE OF ALCOHOL IS A SKULL AND CROSSBONES AND THE WORDS WARNING, POISON.'

Script technique 4: Imagine, and really imagine, that you are now a soldier, vigilant and on constant guard duty, 24/7, watching for the enemy *sugar* trying to enter your body undetected, cunningly disguised as other foods, masquerading as healthy foods; secret sugar, hidden sugar. When sugar enters your stomach it splinters out into millions and billions of little red sugar worms. These little red sugar worms then dangerously damage your body. They slowly destroy your body, attacking from the inside out. Your natural immune system, your home defence, can deal with a small amount but not an infestation. So you will always have to be alert, on guard and very vigilant. You will not allow sugar to enter your body undetected. You will say, "Halt, who goes there? Friend or foe." But always remember that the choice is yours, whether you decide to say, "Welcome, my friend, come in," or, "Please go." NOW imagine the battle between your immune system and the little red sugar worms ending, with your immune system conquering and reigning forever victorious: there can be no other outcome! (This is also a fantastic technique for strengthening your immune system). You have achieved *weight-loss success!* Return to the here and now when the time feels right for you by counting from 1 to 5, then saying, "I'm now wide awake and feeling fine, let battle commence."

*'IMAGINE YOU ARE NOW LOOKING
AND FEELING FANTASTIC!'*

Script technique 5: Imagine, and really imagine, inside your mind is a switch, and above the switch is written *natural instinctive eating* and the switch is in the off position. Now imagine the switch being turned back on just like it was when you were a newborn. This was a time when you ate when you were hungry and stopped when you were satisfied, or, natural instinctive eating. You ate for no reasons other than hunger. For many and various reasons the switch was turned off, but now you have just switched it back on; imagine the switch clicking back on. You are returning back to eating when hungry and stopping when satisfied, just like you did when you were a newborn baby; eating for hunger and nothing else. Your stomach is retracting back to the size nature first decided it should be, not stretched and oversized but the perfect size. You now know it only takes a small amount of food before you feel satisfied. You feel so proud and protective over your stomach that you will not allow it to become stretched and oversized ever again and this feels so good. You have achieved *weight-loss success!* Return to the here and now when the time feels right for you by counting from 1 to 5, then saying, "I'm now wide awake and feeling fine, let battle commence."

When using visualisation it is imperative that you always visualise the things you want and not the thing you have that you really don't want. Always see and transform negatives into positives, destructive into constructive. See yourself kicking all the obstacles out of your life that are responsible for your obesity, because your unconscious mind works on making what you imagine your reality; the objective of M.I.R. visualisation!

Script technique 6: Imagine, and really imagine, that you are, right now, at your natural ideal weight. It's like looking through a mirror into the future, gazing into a crystal ball. See yourself climbing out of bed in the morning and standing in front of a full-length mirror and liking what you see. Imagine the feeling this gives you. Then see yourself standing on the bathroom scales and seeing the weight you always dreamed of being, feel the feeling this gives you. It is a feeling you never want to let go of, a feeling you now know you can very easily achieve, because you really do know that you can be anything you want to be. See yourself on a bright hot sunny day, strolling down the street, dressed in the clothes you want to wear, not the clothes you think you should wear but would otherwise prefer not to. Looking exactly how you want to look, feeling how you want to feel. Other people coming up to you, complimenting you on how strikingly attractive you look, how well and healthy your present appearance is and all because of your *weight-loss success.* You like this feeling, it makes you feel good, really good. You have achieved what others can only dream of achieving. Feel a sense of happiness and pride at your achievement because you now know how easy *weight-loss success* really is – you are a winner. You feel like the cat that's got the cream, a celebrity walking the red carpet. Ten being the highest and zero being the lowest, feel this feeling of happiness and pride as a big 10, because you have now found your utopia. As a hedonist pursues pleasure you have perused and found your own *weight-loss success.* Never show your mind what you don't want, only what you do want, because imagination is the language of the unconscious mind. Show your mind the person you want to be, because what you imagine your unconscious mind will endeavour to make that your ongoing reality. You have achieved *weight-loss success!* Return to the here and now when the time feels right for you by counting from 1 to 5, then saying, "I'm now wide awake and feeling fine, let battle commence."

'A NEW PATTERN OF BEHAVIOUR WITH NO PREDICTABILITY OF EATING.'

Script technique 7: Imagine, and really imagine, your stomach as a factory and running the factory are a work force of hundreds of little workers feeding the metabolism, your engine, with food/fuel to power your body. On the side of your stomach is a great big silver bell. When food/fuel is needed the bell is rung, you will become hungry and food/fuel should be delivered. In the past, you haven't waited for that bell to be rung, have you? You've just continued delivering food/fuel without an order being placed and the foreman of the factory keeps shaking his head, saying, "We have nowhere to put this delivery. It wasn't ordered, and all the storerooms are full to capacity. We'll just have to force more in. Come on, lads, push! We can't send it back, more's the pity!" So the storerooms, your hips, your bum and belly are all bursting full, their walls bulging into all sorts of shapes, but the delivery has to go somewhere as it cannot be returned. To make matters even worse, you just keep making more and more deliveries. You can see what is going to happen, your workforce is working in unacceptable conditions. There's going to be an industrial walkout, a strike, and the factory will one day shut down! Now see the factory functioning harmoniously with all the work force smiling with the storerooms empty and the workers keeping on top of their work because deliveries are only made when the bell is rung. You have achieved *weight-loss success!* Return to the here and now when the time feels right for you by counting from 1 to 5, then saying, "I'm now wide awake and feeling fine, let battle commence."

'YOU WRITE THE STORY.'

Imagine present tense specific things when visualising weight loss. Imagine very detailed aspects of what it will be like to be at your target weight. Think about what it will feel like to have an absence of body fat and a rise in energy. Picture what it will be like to slide easily into a pair of jeans sized for your target weight and how good that will make you feel. Visualise what it will feel like to no longer be out of breath after walking up a flight of stairs, carrying in groceries or chasing the kids around the garden. Imagine the feeling of confidence you will have walking into a social setting whereupon you will be complimented on your new shape and healthy appearance. Knowing you will never have to wear fat-clothes ever again because you will, now, always strive forwards and never drift back. Be creative, write your own stories with you being the star of the show and the whole important happy ever after. Know that this fantasy can become your reality. During visualisation, it's important to maintain an awareness that these fantasies can become real. Having a tiny waistline is not an unrealistic objective for you, remember you can be anything you want to be. Given sufficient time, listening to your body's hunger and satiety signals (natural instinctive eating) and not environmental cues will inevitably lead to weight loss. The purpose of the visualisation technique is to keep your mind focused on the benefits of what life will be like when you achieve your goal and *weight-loss success*. This also makes it less likely that you will stray from making the choices that need to be made in order to achieve your weight loss goal. There are hundreds if not thousands of visualisation scripts available in books, CDs and on the internet, but the best ones are the ones you write yourself as they are more specific and can be targeted at the source of the problem. Become a successful author of your own fairytale, always making sure your story ends with a happy ever after. When you have time write a long story or when you are busy use the 90 second approach. Effective visualisation for *weight-loss success* needn't take up much of your time. Literally, over only the span of about two TV commercials, you can unlock the proven visualisation benefits for your weight loss goals. Spend just 90 seconds per day visualising details of your desired *weight-loss success* as this will give proven results, but the more the better! Top-tip: modern smart phones are fantastic tools for recording scripts to play back through earphones, not a lot of people know that, or do they? Also use a friend or family member to recite them to you.

Mantras, Affirmation or Self-Talk are other very important tools to *weight-loss success*. A mantra, affirmation or self-talk is a conscious word or sentence that you continually repeat in order to remain focused and achieve a goal, as conscious thoughts to bring about desired change. This powerful tool has been used to reach all types of great heights. Many people throughout time have successfully used mantras, affirmations or self-talk in order to lose vast amounts of weight and to feel vibrantly well! Mantras, affirmations or self-talk break up unhealthy or negative patterns that are stored in the unconscious mind. They help us create new, positive ways of thinking that can have amazing results both physically and emotionally. Mantras, affirmations or self-talk are *repetition, repetition, repetition,* use the selection below as well as writing your own, it's fun.

- I can lose weight.
- I deserve to achieve *weight-loss success*.
- I am now confident that I can lose weight and feel fantastic.

- Nothing tastes as good as slim feels.
- I'm slim getting slimmer, I'm fit getting fitter.
- For my life's sake I'm taking control of my plate.
- I can easily and happily achieve my goals.
- One day at a time, I'm looking good and feeling fine.
- I eat only when I'm hungry.
- I stop eating when I'm satisfied.
- I will achieve my natural ideal weight.
- I can be anything I want to be.

Write your own mantras, affirmations or self-talk scripts and use them as much as possible to help you achieve you desired goals and aspirations. The repetition of an action becomes a new learnt behaviour or habitual auto-behaviour. This is something your unconscious mind throughout time has always excelled at. Mantras, affirmations or self-talk are the repetition of your desired goals which, with time and effort, will result in creating and achieving the desired effect: *weight-loss success!*

IMAGINATION IS THE LANGUAGE OF THE UNCONSCIOUS MIND. MIND IMAGERY REPROGRAMMING – M.I.R™ FACILITATES WEIGHT-LOSS SUCCESS!

CHAPTER FIVE

AND FINALLY TO CONCLUDE

The three causes of obesity are *beliefs, behaviours* and *associations.* This correlation has, for far too long, been overlooked when searching for the elusive cure, with food often causing the distraction. We blame genetics, chemical imbalances, big bones and glands, when obesity is a chronic behavioural condition and until treated as such will continue to rampage with great vengeance. Only by the correct information, accurately delivered, will the problem ever be solved.

We have now established that a limiting belief is a belief accepted by the unconscious mind and taken as true or fact based on unreliable, distorted, false and faulty information, which leads to produced actions and associations that stop the individual from reaching their full potential and *weight-loss success.* What most people don't realise is that the vast majority of our beliefs are not really true or fact. Rather, they were accepted long before the critical faculty of the mind was fully formed, thus being denied adequate intellectual analysis and interpretation, along with the imagination playing its key role in the distortion of external information. Breakfast, dinner and tea is such a belief and (to varying degrees) forms the foundations of the condition of human obesity. Through the repetition of an action that is based on a negative limiting belief, detrimental and non-beneficial learnt behaviours or habitual auto-behaviours and corresponding triggered associations form. The end result is the production of beliefs, behaviours and associations, which limits your potential by preventing you from achieving what you, in reality, are truly capable of achieving.

'BREAKFAST, DINNER AND TEA, IS THE ROGUE PROGRAMME THAT LEADS TO MOST, IF NOT ALL, OF THE CONTRIBUTING FACTORS OF HUMAN OBESITY.'

Learnt behaviours or habitual auto-behaviours and corresponding triggered associations are formed from belief. Breakfast, dinner and tea is the rogue programme that leads to most, if not all, of the contributing factors of human obesity. A learnt behaviour or a habitual auto-behaviour is a habit that is performed automatically without conscious intervention with attached associations. We eat breakfast, dinner and tea not because we are hungry, but because it's breakfast-time, dinner-time and tea-time. Eating 'by the clock' interrupts the body's natural regulatory/compensatory system and stops it from working efficiently and effectively. Eating habits born of formed limiting beliefs, such as not leaving the house without having breakfast, is a form of 'Food-Dictation' or 'Predicted eating'. This engenders automated control over what should be an unpredictable and non-dictated response to hunger and satiety signals. Instead of listening to your hunger, these limiting beliefs, behaviours and associations, will allow the clock to trigger food consumption, so you eat at 7.30am (breakfast) 1pm (dinner) and 5.30pm (tea) instead of when hungry. It is this habit that keeps you in a state of obesity. If allowed to go unchanged, these habits will dictate your eating behaviours for the rest of your life. Instigating behavioural change, not food restriction, is the only thing that can lead to *weight-loss success!*

> *'DAILY ACTIONS ARE VAIRABILE, FOOD DICTATION IS PREDICTABLE.'*

J. A. Laundon, 1909-2000

In order to change you life, you have to change your thinking, or cognition, and recognise your limiting beliefs which form the foundations of your learnt behaviours or habitual auto-behaviours and their corresponding triggered associations. By using your inner voice, self-talk or self-chatter, these beliefs, habits and associations can be easily identified and changed – if you *Acknowledge,* you will *Reprogramme* and ultimately *Succeed.* At times you will have conflicts of interest, with your inner voice saying one thing and your unconscious mind saying another. This will be the result of a conflict between what the unconscious mind believes is the true or factual response to a specific situation and what you know consciously is the logical, analytical, reasoned response to the same situation. In these situations we have to make sure that the inner voice of conscious logic shouts back louder than the unconscious mind's limited belief. By using the inner voice of self-chatter we keep mindful and pay conscious attention to the way in which we talk to ourselves, becoming aware and identifying those beliefs that limit our progress. By reprogramming these learnt behaviours or habitual auto-behaviours and adjusting their corresponding triggered associations, through questioning and challenging, you can make the necessary changes to achieve the desired objective, but without identifying them behaviour change cannot take place!

THE SECRET OF TALK YOURSELF SLIM WITH THE SELF-CHATTER DIET

To reignite natural instinctive eating you have to first Acknowledge – ask your inner voice am I hungry or is it something else? Secondly, Reprogramme – respond accordingly to the inner voice's answer. Thirdly, Succeed – the conscious action will change the unconscious programme.

Beliefs, behaviours and associations are the fundamental reasons why we all behave and react in the way we do but at times would otherwise prefer not to, and is so perfectly demonstrated in the state of pregnancy. The expectant mother will start feeding for two and this is a natural response within human development in the gestation period. But here lies the problem, after giving birth the new mum forgets to make the transition back to feeding for one. Before the world evolved into the modern world it is today this transition would have been a natural progression triggered by environment and habitat. In the dramatically modified world of perpetual abundance we have today, these natural triggers no longer have the same impact as they once did, so we have to take the responsibility ourselves. Post-baby weight is becoming an ever-increasing problem and has many psychological and adverse effects on the new mums of today. All this, as if they don't have enough to worry about. By using a smaller plate with smaller portions and serving more if still hungry, by eating at the table without distractions, these tactics will help keep you mindful of the habitual behaviours causing your obesity. Because without recognising negative behaviours, how can behavioural change possibly take place? Don't get weighed every single day as this show a false pattern of your progress due to discrepancies between food eaten and waste excreted. This can, as it so often does, compound a suggestion of failure. And remember, everyone thinks they are a weight loss expert, but these are usually the same people who for whatever reasons cannot control and manage their own weight, so be careful of who you take advice from!

And so to conclude, you, the reader or the solution-seeker, have now been fully armed with an arsenal full of weapons to fight in the battle against obesity. This world is not a perfect place for human existence, as was originally intended, but unfortunately we have no other alternatives. We force feed our children instead of allowing them to feed themselves, creating the cruel effects of childhood obesity. Children should always be fed from tureens and not pre-plated food. We now model our bodies on the images created by the media and regularly fail to recognise the fact that we all have a different genetic make up, even though genetic make up does not dictate obesity. The human prototype was never built from a magazine image. Temptation will always be in the path of *weight-loss success* and the weak will inevitably get waylaid and the strong will always make it to their goal. The original environment in which humans were adapted for survival is long gone. We think we have advanced, but have we? If a world full of obese people is advancement, then yes, we have advanced. We are now feeding on processed foods, which are only depriving the body of trace elements, vitamins and minerals found in fresh primal foods, thus creating disease and demise with a population becoming dependant on pills and potions to counterbalance these effects. This is a fabricated profiteering world, with people being intensively farmed in confined enclosures with a constant supply of feed. Movement has become rare. We are relaying on medication for longevity. Abundance is not always beneficial and food scarcity is not always something we must avoid at all costs. The hunter-gatherer motivation to survive mode is now, detrimentally, seldom used in the modern world in which we all live; that is, eating for hunger/survival and not other environmentally fabricated prompts and cues. If you are true to your word and you have genuine desire to change, I will congratulate you now as *weight-loss success* will be yours. To the rest, I say enjoy to the best of your ability the time you have left, for I sincerely hope the suffering you endure will not be over protracted. This truly comes from the heart, because the answer is here right in front of you now, and it doesn't have to be this way forever!

NATURAL INSTINCTIVE EATING IS LISTENING AND RESPONDING TO THE BODY'S HUNGER AND SATIETY SIGNALS AND NOT FABRICATED ENVIROMENTLE CUES, TO FACILITATE WEIGHT-LOSS SUCCESS!

And as the Yorkshire Poet depicts in his poem, *Be Different, Be You.* You don't have to be like everyone else, you can be different.

BE DIFFERENT, BE YOU

Who says that it's right to wear two matching shoes,
that girls dress in pink and boys dress in blue.
That we must eat breakfast before dinner and dinner
before tea,
who made all of these rules because they didn't ask me.

Take a step out of turn and don't follow the rest,
to do what others expect is not always the best.
Because when you are gone people will say this of you,
here lies a man that's been different, that's true.

From the day that you're born be no one but you,
if people look at you strange it's because they'd like to
do what you do.
For it's too late when you get old to sit down weep,
and cry,
thinking you were born, got married, had children,
then predictably die.

© THE YORKSHIRE POET, 1995

Weight loss experts, medical or not, focus most of their attention on the calorific values of foods, forming an understanding of how and why fat is stored only to produce yet another restrictive diet. Obesity is a behavioural condition, psychological by nature, so restrictive eating has no longevity in the production of a weight loss solution. Until this factor is recognised and generally understood, restrictive diets will only continue to fuel the problem. Without behavioural change nothing will be achieved. By not eating food and only drinking water, weight loss will take place, but for how long can this foolhardy system be maintained and to what degree of damage is being caused? Education has to be directed in the direction of expectorant mothers, preventing the problem before it arises, teaching the method of feeding on demand and the necessity of primal foods and water, as once this is implemented the problem will dramatically reduce; this is nature's way of successful weight management by the *input to expenditure ratio*. We must all return back to the mind-state given at birth to restrain obesity from becoming the catalyst for the mutation of man.

I do hope by now you have discovered the real reason behind the repetition within this book, but even if not, the reason by now will have served its purpose, as truly intended.

The time is here, you are armed and your enemy awaits, let battle commence, and no! This is not just another diet book, but the authentic diet of origin.

DR. ROCKET'S™
**TALK YOURSELF SLIM WITH
THE SELF-CHATTER DIET
'BEHAVIOUR FOCUSED *WEIGHT-LOSS
SUCCESS'***

FOR MORE INFORMATION ON
TREATMENTS,TRAINING, SEMINARS &
CLASSES, OR TO ARANGE A PRIVATE
CONSULTATION AT THE FEELBETTERFAST
'WEIGHT-LOSS' CLINIC, SIMPLY CALL:
07800584077
E-MAIL:
FEELBETTERFAST@BTINTERNET.COM
WEBSITE:
WWW.THESELF-CHATTERDIET.COM

**THE JOURNEY STARTS HERE TO
*WEIGHT-LOSS SUCCESS… THE EASY WAY!***

*JOHN RICHARDSON – BEHAVIOURAL
WEIGHT-LOSS CONSULTANT / NBW-LP*
IN ASSOCIATION WITH THE NATIONAL
BEHAVIOURAL WEIGHT-LOSS PROGRAMME
& THE FEELBETTERFAST CLINIC

TRAIN AND BECOME A BEHAVIOURAL
WEIGHT-LOSS CONSULTANT AND CLASS
FACILITATOR EARNING THE DISTINCTION
Dip: NBW-LP/S-CD. FIRST CLASS TRAINING
WILL BE GIVEN IN THE SYSTEMATIC
METHOD OF, TALK YOURSELF SLIM WITH
THE SELF-CHATTER DIET, FOCUSING ON
BEHAVIOURAL CHANGE LEADING TO
WEIGHT-LOSS SUCCESS!

On completion of the course you will have gained a full understanding of the behavioural psychology that leads to obesity, along with the capability and competence to successfully help clients achieve *weight-loss success*. Once the required levels of theory comprehension and practical implementation has been achieved you will be entitle to become a 'Behavioural Weight-Loss Consultant' and 'Class Facilitator' for *Dr. Rocket's Talk Yourself Slim With The Self-Chatter Diet,* organising and running your own behaviour focused weight-loss classes, along with private consultations facilitating *weight-loss success,* with all the help and support of The National Behavioural Weight-Loss Programme (NBW-LP) & The Feelbetterfast Clinic. For more information call: 07800584077 or visit the website:

WWW.THESELF-CHATTERDIET.COM

JOHN RICHARDSON – BEHAVIOURAL
WEIGHT-LOSS CONSULTANT / NBW-LP
**IN ASSOCIATION WITH THE NATIONAL
BEHAVIOURAL WEIGHT-LOSS
PROGRAMME & THE FEELBETTERFAST
CLINIC**

**WATCH OUT FOR A CLASS, CONSULTANT
OR SEMINAR NEAR YOU!**

**TALK YOURSELF SLIM WITH
THE SELF-CHATTER DIET,
PROVIDING 'THE ANSWER' TO
WEIGHT LOSS SUCCESS**

**'AS ONE THING ENDS SOMETHING
NEW BEGINS'**

John Richardson